THE ACNE SOLUTION

Breakthroughs in Treating Acne
That Will Work for You!

ZEEV PAM M.D., SHMUEL YORAV M.D.

ZEEV PAM M.D. | SHMUEL YORAV M.D.

THE ACNE SOLUTION
BREAKTHROUGHS IN TREATING ACNE
THAT WILL WORK FOR YOU!

Translators: Zeev Pam M.D. and Shmuel Yorav M.D.

Editor: Sherrill Layton

Illustration: Mira Fridman

Cover: Benjie Herskowitz

Layout Design: Sergey Desyatkov

ISBN: 978-1-59120-382-7

This book is dedicated in loving memory to our co-author,
Dr. Zeev Pam, an outstanding Israeli dermatologist.
(1953-2013)

Dr. Zeev Pam was an exceptionally smart, humble, and
kind person. He was a great example to all the people
around him both professionally and personally. He passed
away while this book was being prepared
for production in English.

He will be forever loved, missed, and remembered by his
family, friends, colleagues, patients, and readers.

Acknowledgments

Dr. Yorav

To my two sons, **Roy and On Yorav**; and special thanks goes to my wife, **Orna Yorav**, for her great dedication to this project.

We owe thanks to **Dr. Yoram Harth** for his enlightening information on phototherapy;

and to **Dr. Nadav Pam** for his contribution in reference to food and its influence on acne;

Dr. Zeev Pam

To my beloved wife Sara Pam and two sons Ori and Nadav Pam

PREFACE

A quick peek into a dermatologist's crowded clinic is enough to make us realize that acne is no small matter. For most of the adolescents filling the waiting rooms, the pimples on their skin are insufferable, truly the "end of the world." Every zit on the face, back or chest becomes the main, and sometimes the only, thing in their lives. Every glance in the mirror is accompanied by severe frustration and anger: Why me? Why now, of all times?

One can easily empathize with the emotions arising in teenagers upon the eruption of pimples, given that they usually first appear at the most beautiful time of our youth:

It happens at the worst time. Just when you are slowly forming your own identity and finding your place in society. Exactly when you are so conscious of your appearance and wish to look your very best. And just now, of all times, these pimples appear all over your skin making you feel unattractive and threatening to rob you of a good chunk of your self-confidence.

Acne does not always disappear at the end of adolescence. Quite a few adults still bear this condition from their youth, while some others only begin to develop acne in adulthood.

Quite gloomy thus far... Fortunately, together with the bad news, there is also good news. Great breakthroughs in treating acne have been made in recent years; new and successful treatment methods have been developed, and today—much more than in the past—medical professionals can offer real help to sufferers.

We, who encounter thousands of concerned adolescents in the course of our work, know how difficult a time this is. Therefore, we decided to invite you to join us on a "what it's all about" tour of acne. The following pages explain what is happening on and under the skin, and the full range of acne treatments.

This book is meant for adolescents, and is also suitable for their parents so that they can participate in the process their children are going through, as well as for adults who suffer from this disorder. It is intended to also serve as a guide for cosmeticians, pharmacists, nurses, doctors, and all those who want and need to understand the real story of acne.

Table of Contents

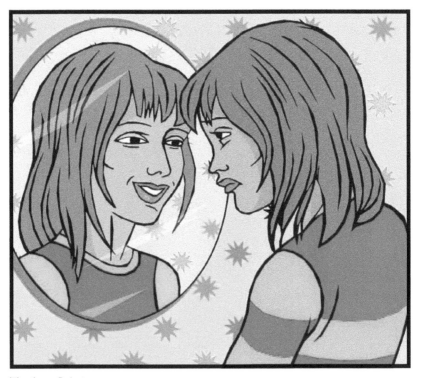

The Acne Solution –

Chapter 1

CLEARING THE FOG SURROUNDING ACNE

You're right! Knowing about the structure of the skin and understanding the causes of acne is not essential for treating this disorder. You can do so without it. In fact, you can skip this chapter altogether, go directly to the more advanced chapters and find the answers to questions that bother you: How to treat the inflamed pimples, what preparations are suitable for treating blackheads and whiteheads, or what factors aggravate them.

We believe, though, that by becoming acquainted with the processes that hasten the eruption of that new pimple that popped up on your face this morning, you'll be better able to prevent, as much as possible, the appearance of more pimples.

Even more, knowing the terms used by skin doctors will improve the cooperation between you and your doctor and will result in faster and more successful treatment.

LOOKING INSIDE

Most of us think of our skin as just the part of the body that separates us from the external world, nothing more. In fact, the skin — the largest organ of the body — is not just some big bag in which we are wrapped. It is an organ composed of billions of cells and it remains active nonstop: it protects us from invasions by bacteria, removes waste products through its pores, serves as the body's heat regulator, transmits messages from the surroundings to our brain, and provides us with the enjoyable sensations of living. The skin is in a constant state of creation and destruction; new cells are being born while, at the same time, old cells die. The outer skin layer is constantly replacing its cells. Just try to think about this: every minute the skin sheds 250,000 dead cells, and it completely replaces itself every 28 days!

The entire surface of the skin, except for the inside of our hands and the bottom of our feet, is covered with small dimples containing hair follicles — channels through which the hair travels on the way to the skin surface. In most parts of the body, the hair is so fine and thin that it is almost invisible. In some areas of the body, the hair never rises above the skin surface, while in others the hair is thicker and longer, as well as more prominent and visible.

Three-Act Play

Skin is composed of three layers, each of which is made up of additional minute layers. The innermost layer of the skin is **subcutaneous tissue** consisting of fatty cells. It forms a sort of padded partition between the internal parts of the body and the two outer skin layers, which it also supports.

On top of this fatty layer is the **dermis** layer, containing a fibrous base that gives skin its flexibility, networks of blood vessels, sweat glands, nerve endings, hair follicles and sebaceous glands. **Hair**

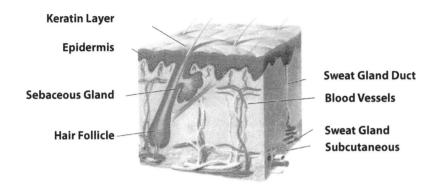

Keratin Layer

Epidermis

Sebaceous Gland

Hair Follicle

Sweat Gland Duct

Blood Vessels

Sweat Gland

Subcutaneous

follicles are minute channels through which the hair grows. **Sebaceous glands** are attached to and open to the hair follicles, lubricating both the hair and the skin.

The external layer, what we see every morning in our mirror, is the **epidermis**. If you look at it through a microscope, it'll appear rough and coarse due to the dead skin cells collecting on the surface before they shed.

It is truly astonishing to discover how thin this outer layer of epidermis that protects our skin is. Its thickness is a mere 0.015mm. (The bottoms of our feet and our inner palms are covered with a thicker layer, about half a millimeter.) The epidermis layer also contains **melanin** cells, which give skin its color.

Acne: What Went Wrong?

A disorder with many causes, the basic, primary cause of acne is not completely clear. What we do know is that three main factors are involved:

Increased production of sebum (skin oil), clogged hair follicles, and excessive multiplication of bacteria. Let's try to understand how each of these affects the eruption of acne.

First of all: Hormones and Adolescence

Hormones are mediating chemical substances produced by the body that regulate almost all body functions. Puberty begins when the pituitary gland, located at the base of the brain, signals the body to begin producing sex hormones. In women, two sex hormones, estrogen and progesterone, are produced in the ovaries.

In men, the sex hormone testosterone is produced in the testes. Progesterone and testosterone are very similar chemically, and they belong to the same class of hormones known as androgens.

Sebaceous Glands Never Rest

The transition from childhood to adolescence is a time of profound adjustment for the body. Suddenly swamped with very powerful androgen hormones, the system can easily overreact to the intensified stimulus. Sebaceous glands respond by increasing sebum production way beyond the normal amount needed to lubricate the skin and hair, and the excess oil overloads the sebaceous ducts and the hair follicles.

Tests have shown that hormone levels of most acne sufferers are normal, and not any higher than of those who don't suffer from the disorder, as is commonly believed. It works the other way around, as well: some people with very high androgen levels sprout no more than a pimple or two. So it would seem that it is the sebaceous gland and its sensitivity to the hormonal stimulus that affects the outbreak of acne.

Just as the sensitivity of the sebaceous glands varies from one person to another, it also varies in the different parts of our bodies. One person may suffer from an eruption of acne on the face, but not on the back or chest, even though the density of sebaceous glands in all three areas is very high (nearly 10,000 just on the dermis layer of the face!).

The Hair Follicle: A Clogged Drain

You'll recall that dead skin cells accumulate in the outer skin layer, giving the skin its protective cover. A similar accumulation of cells also takes place in the pores of the skin. But while the cells on the surface are easily replaced each day, those hidden in the hair follicle need to be flushed out by a stream of sebum.

On their way up to the skin surface, the cells manufacture a coarse hornlike protein called **keratin.** (Remember this term. Keratin plays a very important role in the formation of acne and we'll deal with it later in the book.)

At times the process in the hair follicle space goes awry. Thousands of dead skin cells — loaded with keratin — adhere to each other, together with sebum, hair remnants and bacteria and their products, forming a plug in the hair follicle. And if this isn't enough, for some reason not yet completely clear, the production of skin cells is speeded up. Now more and more cells collect in the hair follicle, contributing to the rapid buildup of the keratin plug.

The keratin plug causes vast amounts of sebum — manufactured, you will recall, in increased amounts — to be trapped in the hair follicle channel so that only a small part of it gets out to the surface. So now, the ground has been prepared for the development of blackheads and whiteheads and non-inflammatory pimples — this marks the point of departure for acne.

When bacteria join the process, as we will soon see, things get worse. Bacteria contribute to the more serious type of inflammatory acne.

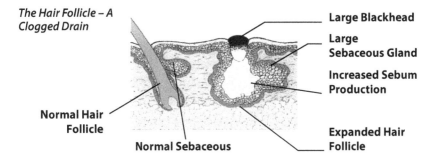

The Hair Follicle – A Clogged Drain

Large Blackhead

Large Sebaceous Gland

Increased Sebum Production

Normal Hair Follicle

Normal Sebaceous

Expanded Hair Follicle

Bacteria: Get them while they're small

The bad name pinned on germs as causes of diseases isn't always justified: Among these tiny creatures are many beneficial bacteria fulfilling various functions. However, we'll see in this example that a surplus of beneficial bacteria can also cause us harm (sort of too much of a good thing).

Many bacteria on the skin surface protect it from invasions of evil-minded bacteria. One of these is a tiny creature with a long name: *Propionibacterium acnes* (p. acnes). This bacterium feeds on the sebum secreted onto the skin. With surplus sebum available on skin that is inclined toward acne, the bacteria is encouraged to multiply excessively: A true population explosion.

WHY DID I GET IT?

Heredity and a Bit of Luck

Many of you probably ask, why me? Why did I get it? Why do my friends get a pimple here, another there, that disappear without a trace, while my face is covered with so many zits, so hard to treat, and for so long? Indeed, this is one of the mysteries of acne. Scientists and researchers don't know precisely why acne develops on a particular skin and not on another. It is believed that heredity plays an important role in the outbreak of the disorder. If one or both of your parents suffered from acne, it is likely that you will suffer from it as well. Apparently, what is inherited is the high sensitivity of the sebaceous glands to the hormonal stimulus.

FACE IN THE MIRROR

Having pimples on your face, you most likely also examine the faces of your companions in misery and quickly discover that each has his/her own type of pimples: Some have pimples that are all of the same type, while others have a mixture of different types. Not only that, but different types of pimples can appear on the same face at different times.

Now the time has come to become acquainted with the whole range of afflictions typical of the disorder — from the minor to the troublesome:

Blackheads

Contrary to common belief, these blackheads, found mostly around the nose, cheeks and chin, are not caused by dirt. It is the fatty plug of the hair follicle that causes the blackhead. When the plug reaches the skin surface, it is exposed to air, oxidizes, and turns black.

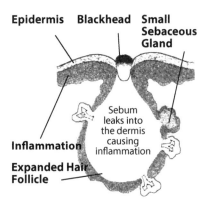

Whiteheads

A whitehead is a closed fatty plug. It appears as a small white or skin colored bump right under the skin. Some whiteheads disappear by themselves, but others are tiny "time bombs." After a while, they grow, stretching the walls of the hair follicle until they burst, releasing their contents into the surrounding skin tissue, and causing an inflammation in the form of a reddish papule.

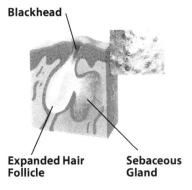

(Dermatologists and other professionals term both blackheads and whiteheads as "comedones.")

Papules

A papule (or as we refer to it, "pimple") is a small red inflamed bump. The sebum that spills out from the whitehead into the surrounding tissue triggers a defensive response by our body whenever it identifies a foreign object. It then immediately sends white blood cells to the affected area, which fight the intruders, leading to swelling and redness. The redness of the pimple also means that the sebum is irritating the skin tissue surrounding the pimple.

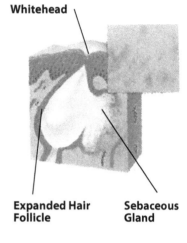

Whitehead

Expanded Hair Follicle   **Sebaceous Gland**

Pustules

In the presence of nearby bacteria, the papules turn into pustules (a lesion or a blister containing pus-filled fluid). This is a much more serious form of acne, indicating infection. The bacteria feed on the surplus sebum and multiply, in the course of which they interfere with the normal functioning of the skin. In reaction, the body sends to the afflicted area an entire army of white cells to fight off the invaders.

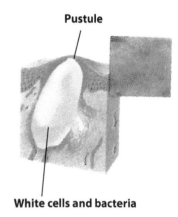

Pustule

White cells and bacteria

Cysts

The most serious stage in the development of the inflammatory process is
a large red lesion forming deep under
the skin. It may be painful and may last
what seems to be forever.

A cyst is formed when the pore is
completely plugged. The secreted sebum
collects and is pushed deeper into the
sebaceous gland, causing it to expand
until a mass is formed that pushes the
skin surface outward. Cysts are considered a serious problem, as they may leave
scars on the skin.

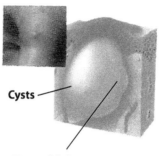

Cysts

Normal Sebaceous

SOME FACTS YOU OUGHT TO KNOW:

Over 80% of the population suffers from acne at some stage of their lives, mostly in adolescence.

Frequency of acne is identical in men and women, but men suffer the more severe forms of the disorder.

Peak frequency: Girls aged 14-17 and boys aged 16-19. The disorder usually fades by itself in the third decade of life.

In 10% of the cases, primarily among women, acne persists even beyond the age of 30.

In up to 10% of women, acne first appears in their 20s and 30s.

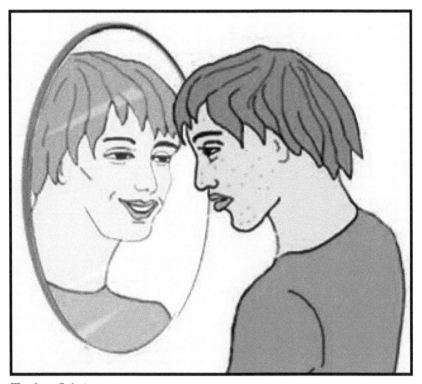

The Acne Solution –

Chapter 2

TRUE OR FALSE? DEMOLISHING MYTHS

As if the pimples erupting on your skin aren't enough, the many myths about acne, almost all of which point an accusing finger at you, plague you: this all happened because you're stuffing yourself with chocolate, or because you're not carefully cleaning your face, or because you're not having sex!

Let's keep in mind that acne is a skin disorder affected by hormonal processes in the body. It is neither caused by something that you do nor by something that you don't do. While it sometimes may get worse due to exposure to certain substances, and may erupt again as a result of taking specific drugs or using certain cosmetics (about all that in the next chapter), it is, in most cases, not related to external causes.

Let's examine each myth. Some are based on facts, while others are clearly false.

Only Teenagers Suffer from Acne

FALSE! | Although most of those suffering from acne are adolescents, they are by no means alone.

Pimples disappear by themselves within a few years in 70% of teenage cases, but may persist on the faces of the other 30% for quite some time beyond adolescence, into the thirties and even longer.

Acne in adulthood is not necessarily a "leftover" of adolescent pimples. It can even strike adults who never had a single pimple as teenagers.

Even newborn babies may suffer from acne due to hormones present in their mother's milk. Such acne usually passes within a few months after nursing ends, and requires no special treatment.

Acne is Caused by Consumption of Fats and Chocolate

FALSE! | While no connection is known to exist between eating certain foods and the outbreak of pimples, this is the most common myth among teenagers as well as their parents. Many are convinced that eating certain foods aggravates or even causes acne. In the last decade, more scientific evidence about the connection between diary food and acne has come to light. The cause is the androgenic hormones found in milk.

The reason is that milk and other dairy products are a major milestone in the human diet.

The combination of morning cereals that include milk and sugar is also very common in human nutrition. The sugar has an additive effect to androgens in milk that can provoke acne. The sugar can influence acne due to insulin metabolism. The sugar can cause high levels of insulin in the blood. This effect for long periods can have an androgenic effect on the skin.

In obese women with hormonal problems, the androgenic effect of milk and sugar might be even worse.

There is no comment against consuming dairy food, but it is worthwhile in some cases to stop or diminish the use of dairy food for 3-4 weeks. This can improve acne treatment in 2% of the patients.

Many families discuss at length what foods to eat or not to eat, and take less interest in medical treatment. In most instances fault is attributed to foods like chocolate, nuts and fries. Chocolate on its own does not aggravate acne. However, the high concentration of sugar in it, might play a role in aggravating acne.

Foods that include high amounts of carbohydrates like pastry, cakes, hard cheeses, ice cream, white flower, pizza, and soft drink rich in sugar, sometimes worsen androgenic acne by inducing a hyperglycemic effect.

How did it come about that nutrition took center stage as the culprit responsible for all acne disorders? We don't know. What we do know is that not enough research has been done on this, mostly because it is so difficult to isolate the nutrition components of all the variables related to our lifestyles and body processes. The few studies that have been conducted rejected any connection between acne and eating chocolate or fatty foods.

The Exceptions

TRUE! Still, there are those who state with certainty – and they may be right – that they experience a direct and immediate connection between eating a particular food and the pimple that pops up the next day.

For those people, we can suggest several solutions:

• If pimples erupt on your face a day, or even a few days or so after you attacked and devoured that chocolate bar, don't look at it as direct proof of a connection between the two. It could be that another factor is lurking in the background, such as emotional stress. In which case it is almost certain that this is what is driving you to the cookie jar and causes the onset of acne.

• Every person has a different sensitivity threshold, due to many factors. So, even without scientific proof, it is quite possible that a certain food may encourage the appearance of pimples in some people, while the skin of others (who stuff themselves with that very same food), remains infuriatingly clear.

If you believe that a particular food hastens the eruption of pimples on your skin, you can try a simple experiment. Try not eating it for two weeks and see if your skin condition improves during that time. If it improves, don't simply rush to give up this food totally and forever. It may be worthwhile to give it another trial period.

A Balanced Diet is Good for Your Health

As a rule, a balanced diet is recommended both for the clear skinned and the pimpled. The general condition of the body is important, because a healthy body can fight acne more easily. If you're not sure that your daily diet is well-balanced, go to a dietician for advice and choose an eating plan that is right for you.

Obese and Diabetic Persons Suffer More from Acne

FALSE! | Many believe that people who are overweight, are diabetics, or have high blood fat levels, are more likely to suffer from acne, but it is not so. It could be that this is connected to a belief (mistaken as well) that there is a link between high-calorie/high-fat (hyperglycemic effect) foods and acne.

Whatever the case, medical studies show that sufferers from diabetes, including juvenile diabetes, or those with high blood fat levels, do not suffer more from acne than the rest of the population

Not Having Sex Causes Acne

FALSE! | You're not alone in thinking so: This conjecture is often whispered in the ear of the physician treating adolescents. It's not hard to understand how this myth developed. Exactly at the age when you start taking an interest in sex, pimples pop up. But, it's just a coincidence, nothing more. In fact, there is no connection whatsoever between the appearance of acne and thoughts of sex, having sex or masturbation. Although acne is caused by the action of hormones on the sebaceous gland, it is not affected by sexual activity.

With all this, having age-appropriate sex may relieve mental stress, and this, just by the way, may improve the appearance of your skin.

Frequent Cleansing of the Skin Prevents Acne

FALSE! | Acne is not caused by dirt.
Many think otherwise. They scrub the pimples covering their face and use every soap and cleaning product they

can think of. In fact, excessive cleaning has very little effect on the state of the acne, except maybe making it worse. Proper hygiene is good for all of us, but its absence does not cause pimples. Washing the face with cleansing substances several times a day dries out the upper skin layer, and may even make it oversensitive to the preparations for treating acne.

The right way to keep skin clean is explained at length in *Chapter 5*. Here we would only like to mention that washing the face twice a day with a suitable soap, the kind that doesn't contain substances that encourage acne, is highly recommended. For those with delicate and sensitive skin, specific cleaning preparations are needed, with special caution to be taken to avoid rough scrubbing of the skin.

Acne Improves During Pregnancy

FALSE! There's no way of predicting how pregnancy will affect acne. Some women claim that their acne improves during the months of pregnancy, while others complain that the condition is aggravated. There are even those who first develop acne during this period.

Improvement in the condition of pimples in some women is apparently related to the higher level of female hormone during pregnancy, which suppresses the action of the male hormone, and reduces its effect on the formation of acne. Of course, pregnancy is not one of the recommended treatments for acne!

What is important during pregnancy, is to exercise great caution when taking medicinal preparations for treatment of acne (*see Chapter 10*).

Acne Can Go Away by Itself

TRUE! BUT... In many cases, acne really does go away by itself without any treatment at all, but this is something that can't be taken for granted.

While 70% percent of youngsters who suffer from acne are indeed cured without any treatment within 4-5 years, for many this period seems longer than eternity. They suffer greatly from the facial pimples and they also may be left with permanent scarring, not to mention the social and emotional difficulties, all during what are supposed to be the best years of their lives.

Even more serious is the situation of the 30% that do not recover within this period, with acne remaining with them for many long years.

To stop the process before it gets out of control, and to prevent further damage, it is very important to begin the treatment as son as possible. Why suffer for no reason at all?

"Popping" Pustules is Harmless

FALSE! | Drive this into your head again and again: Popping zits is strictly prohibited! Popping pustules with your fingers may cause serious damage to the skin. While you may succeed in ejecting the contents of the pimple by squeezing the skin, you will also damage the internal structure of the sebaceous gland and the hair follicle, increase the risk of inflammation, and open the way to the formation of a scar.

In every case, it is important to treat the pimple according to the doctor's instructions and reduce the risk of scarring.

Exposure to the Sun Relieves Acne

TRUE BUT NOT RECOMMENDED! | Risk of damage to the skin from exposure to solar radiation is far greater than the expected benefit. Although sun dries the pimples and perhaps promotes their healing, ultraviolet radiation may promote cancerous processes and hasten aging of the skin.

For these reasons, this treatment method is absolutely not recommended, except for especially difficult cases of acne, and even then exposure to the sun should only be practiced in a controlled and careful manner under medical supervision.

The same goes for artificial tanning in a solarium or by a quartz lamp. In *Chapter 5*, you'll read about an innovative treatment method based on the principle of the blue rays in sunlight.

Brewer's Yeast is a Beneficial Treatment for Acne

FALSE! Brewer's yeast is ordinary baker's yeast, containing 50% protein and a high concentration of vitamin B-complex, niacin, and folic acid.

However, contrary to common belief, brewer's yeast has little effect on acne.

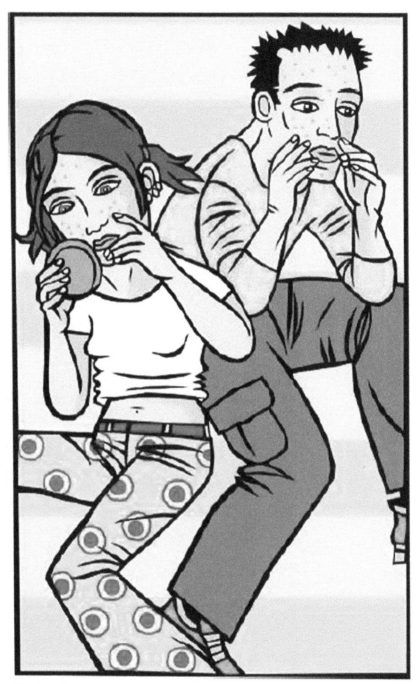

The Acne Solution –

Chapter 3
WHAT AGGRAVATES ACNE?

There are factors that may aggravate acne, some of which are even known to actually cause the disorder. Avoiding these as much as possible may contribute greatly to the health of your skin.

HORMONES

Female Hormones

When it comes to women, several possible reasons may account for changes in hormone levels: Going on or off birth control pills, the menstrual period, or hormonal disorders such as Polycystic Ovary Syndrome (PCOS). All these may aggravate acne.

Birth Control Pills

The two types of oral contraceptives in use are a combined pill containing two female hormones, estrogen and progesterone, and another which contains only progesterone. Estrogen is considered to be "acne-friendly," as it reduces the effect that the male hormone (testosterone) has on the development of acne, and in turn reduces the severity of pimples. Progesterone, on the other hand, can break down in the liver and produce a hormone similar to testosterone, which could aggravate the condition.

So if you are using birth control pills, it is very important to ask your gynecologist to find you a pill that will also enhance the treatment of your acne.

Menstrual Period

Many girls and women experience a sudden outbreak of pimples a number of days before their period, usually just a few erupting on the chin, forehead, and cheeks.

Such flare-ups are very common and simply explained: Just before the menses, the estrogen level drops and the progesterone level rises, opening the way for more pimples. These usually disappear by themselves within a few days without any treatment whatsoever.

Polycystic Ovary Syndrome

Polycystic Ovary Syndrome (PCOS), like its name, is a condition where many small cysts (liquid-filled "pockets") develop in the ovaries. The syndrome manifests itself in many ways, including as acne.

Girls and women who suffer from severe acne that does not respond well to treatment, and who also experience excessive hairiness or irregular periods, are usually sent for tests to determine if they are suffering from this syndrome.

The common treatment for PCOS is Diane 35 (birth control pill), sometimes together with Androcur. Both pills contain cyproterone acetate, a unique ingredient that reduces the effect of the male hormone testosterone on the sebaceous glands and prevents their hyperactivity. Using these medications is also helpful in treating other PCOS syndrome-related problems.

Male Hormones – Anabolic Steroids

If you're working hard to build up your muscles and taking anabolic steroids (artificial male hormone additive), listen up! Using these preparations may affect activity of the sebaceous glands and lead to a severe outbreak of acne, even among men who have never suffered from pimples. This eruption, in the form of red pimples with or without pus, but without blackheads or whiteheads, appears just a few days after beginning steroids, and usually disappears on its own after stopping.

STRESS

Constant stress aggravates many skin problems, and certainly acne. Most of you are well aware of this from personal experience. Studies also indicate a link between conditions of stress and tension and outbreaks of acne.

No one is immune to the effects of stress on the body: each person has his own weak link. If you suffer from acne, your body's weak link may be the sebaceous glands, and when you're stressed out, it will focus there.

Vicious Cycle: Stress, Acne, and... Stress

Most of us live and function in an environment characterized by a great deal of stress and tension. At various times in our lives we cope with stress related to studies, social situations, careers and making a living, marriage, and bringing up children. At times the tension is so intense and so prolonged that it appears to us to be the norm that this is how things should be.

Increased tension aggravates acne, often creating a vicious cycle. As the pimples continue to take over your skin, especially your face, you're just a short step away from feelings of inferiority, anxiety and depression, which so often, particularly in adolescence, can lead to social isolation. This situation in turn creates tremendous stress that contributes to—you've already guessed—an aggravation of acne.

Shocks to Hormone Functions

When we're stressed out, certain hormonal changes which originate in the adrenal glands take place in our body. These two tiny glands perched on our kidneys produce many hormones, some of which stimulate increased activity of the sebaceous glands. In times of stress, the sebaceous glands work nonstop and cause the formation of more pimples.

Weakening of the Immune System

Stress and tension also reduce the body's resistance to bacteria by weakening the effectiveness of the immune system. This leaves us not only more exposed to colds and other infectious diseases, but an outbreak of acne can be expected as well.

"Out-Stress" the Stress

A certain amount of stress is essential and even healthy. Functioning under stress can improve creativity and contribute to finding creative solutions to problems. The question is how to reduce the stress level so that you can enjoy its benefits without harming your bodily and mental health?

First of all, you must learn to identify the stress and tension which affect you and recognize the close links to pimples on your skin. Only after you work through this stage will you be able to seek out the various techniques for reducing stress and gaining real benefits.

Reducing stress and releasing tension can be accomplished in several ways, such as:
- Regular and continuous physical activity
- Getting enough sleep
- Balanced menu and avoiding stimulants such as caffeine
- Relaxation through methods such as yoga, meditation, and proper breathing exercises
- Sharing your problems with others. Hiding tension only makes it worse. Better to talk and consult with friends or professionals

PICKING PIMPLES

A direct cause of aggravating acne. Never pick or squeeze pimples! Squeezing spreads the inflammation and with time increases the risk of scarring.

COSMETIC PRODUCTS

Skin care is dealt with in full in *Chapter 5*. We would only like to note here that it is recommended that all skin care and cosmetic products be treated with caution. Ointments and creams, rouge and lipstick, eye shadow, moisturizing cream and sunscreen; all these may cause acne or contribute to its worsening. Using oil-based gel on your hair may also lead to pimples, particularly on the forehead and the sides of the face that make contact with hair.

Most victims of cosmetic products are women in their twenties to forties, who suffered from acne in their youth. The process of curing this type of acne is usually quite slow, and it is common for the pimples to persist long after product use is discontinued.

This, however, doesn't mean you should avoid cosmetic products. They can be of great benefit in hiding or blurring pimples and improving your feelings and self-confidence. Just check them out before you buy them and make certain they are acne-friendly, that they come from a reputable source, and have not been slapped together by amateurs.

Most cosmetic products manufactured by respectable companies are thoroughly tested to ensure that they do not clog pores, causing blackheads or whiteheads. Recommended products are usually marked "non-comedogenic" or "oil-free."

MEDICATIONS

Certain medications may cause acne or aggravate existing pimples. It is most important that you know this: if you are suffering from acne and taking one of the drugs mentioned in this section, consult with your physician and ask him to prescribe, if possible, an alternative medication that does not have the same side effects.

The principal drugs that cause a rash similar to acne, or that aggravate existing acne, are of the steroid family:

Corticosteroids – These substances are found in many medications used for treating inflammatory skin diseases, allergies, illnesses in which the immune system is involved, malignant disorders, and in preventing transplant rejection.

Anabolic and Androgen Steroids – Artificial addition of male hormones for building up body muscle.

The female **progesterone** hormone, used in birth control pills, may also aggravate acne.

Additional medication groups that cause acne:

Hydantoin and Phenobarbitone – Medications for treating epilepsy

Lithium – For treating manic-depression

Isoniazid and Rifampicin – For treatment of tuberculosis

Iodides and Bromides (halogens) – Used in tranquilizers, cough syrups and vitamins

Anesthetics – Chloral hydrate and halothane

Others – Quinine, sulfur, psoralen + UVA, thiouracil, disulfiram, thiourea. These medications are not a frequent cause of acne.

OCCUPATION

Exposure to certain substances at work, or certain work conditions, may cause the appearance of pimples or aggravate existing pimples.

Here are some typical examples of risk groups:

- Working around fuel and oil: mechanics, gas station attendants, operators of oil-cooled cutting machines, road paving workers, etc.
- Working around halogens (particularly chlorine): woodworking industry workers, workers with pesticides, in manufacturing of preservative materials and in the chemical and pharmaceutical industries
- Prolonged and permanent use of cosmetic preparations: actors, models, beauty consultants, TV moderators, etc.
- Activity involving prolonged chafing of body areas such as the back and buttocks, or always wearing very tight clothing—risk groups: drivers, athletes, and others

TEMPERATURE, PERSPIRATION, AND HUMIDITY

Temperature

As temperature rises, the rate of production of sebum in the skin pores increases. This is the reason that in the summer heat many people sense that their skin is oily, while those who suffer from acne discover that their condition worsens.

If you are light skinned, it would be best to be particularly wary of exposure to the sun, not only because of the UV radiation, but also because in rare cases your skin may react by erupting in red pimples over the shoulders, arms, neck and chest.

Perspiration and High Humidity

One of the main reasons for the development of acne is the accumulation of dead skin cells that partially plug the hair duct. In a humid environment, when perspiration collects on the skin surface, the dead cells absorb large amounts of moisture, swell rapidly, and aggravate the clogging of hair follicles.

In hot and humid seasons, acne rashes can appear in various degrees of severity, primarily among those engaged in vigorous physical activity at work or in their hobbies. Typically, the rashes appear mostly on the back, chest, buttocks and hips, and less on the face.

ACNE AND NUTRITION
IN A NUTSHELL

On the Link Between Acne and Nutritional Ingredients

The link between the appearance of acne and various nutritional ingredients is a very common assumption. Most adolescents and their parents are convinced that eating certain foods such as chocolate, nuts, donuts, hard cheese, and others, cause acne.

The reason for assuming there is a link between acne and nutrition, particularly sweets, peanuts, almonds, sunflower seeds and pistachio nuts, is not clear as yet; although it would be logical to connect fatty foods to increased production of sebum in the skin. From here, one could project that if rich foods are consumed, there is increased production of fat from the sebaceous glands in the skin, leading to the development of acne.

However, assumptions have thus far no scientific or research basis whatsoever in the medical world. Comparative tests of the composition of sebum and oils produced on the skin surface showed no similarity to the ingredients of ingested high-fat food.

How Do Fats and Sugars in Food Affect the Formation of Acne?

There are two schools of thought. Some argue that sugars and fats in food may serve as a store of energy for the bacteria in the skin's sebaceous glands. Food additives, androgen-like hormones (testosterone), as well as salts and other food additives, could lead to the formation of acne.

Some food additives and vitamins also contain salts and halogens (cooking salt, iodine, chlorine, bromine) as part of their manufacturing process. Their absorption into the blood and discharge through the sebaceous glands stimulates the glands to increase sebum production.

In this era of industrialized agriculture, we employ pesticides, fertilizers, recycled feed, and medications in the process of producing food from plants and animals, some of which are hormonal.

So when we consume fresh or preserved food, even if the health authorities have approved it, we cannot know how, and with what substances, the food was treated, and at times we become unwittingly exposed to ingredients that could cause acne.

Conclusion: We need to examine the contents of the food that we buy, and avoid certain food ingredients.

Against the theory that there is a connection between acne and nutrition, opponents argue that the principal bodily changes in adolescence are hormonal and not dependent on nutrition. Offered as proof is the fact that vegetarians and naturalists suffer from acne at a rate similar to that of the general population, while diabetics or those with high blood fat do not suffer from acne more than healthy people do.

Even though most physicians do not link acne and nutrition, consulting with nutrition professionals should be considered when and if necessary.

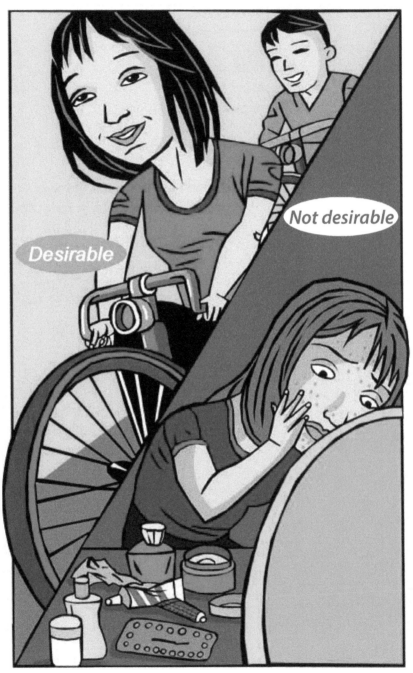

The Acne Solution –

Chapter 4

TREATING ACNE –
ONE STEP AT A TIME

Once it was believed that acne did not have to be treated, since in most cases it would go away by itself. Now we know that proper treatment given in time can prevent acne from getting worse and reduces the risk of scarring – physical as well as mental.

Treatment of acne is complicated and determined by the severity of the pimples of each and every person.

How severe is your personal acne problem? How can you tell? How to swim through an entire ocean of "Grandma's remedies" and advice and stories from your friends and come up with the treatment that is best suited for you? How to decide at what stage to go to a doctor? What awaits you at each and every stage?

Let us now try to guide you through all this, one step at a time.

HOW SEVERE IS YOUR ACNE?

Our review of acne treatments in the coming chapters is arranged by type of treatment and according to severity of the acne. Look carefully at your face in the mirror and use the definitions below to grade your acne.

You, of course, are the one who will decide whether to treat the pimples by yourself or go for professional treatment. But you should know that each person needs an individually prepared course of treatment, tailored exactly to her/his needs, according to the type of acne, its severity, type of skin and general health.

PHARMACIST, COSMETICIAN, OR DERMATOLOGIST

By Yourself
Advised by a Pharmacist or Cosmetician

If your acne is very mild, the first place you visit will most likely be the pharmacy to seek the assistance of the pharmacist. You should keep in mind that there are many active substances for treating acne on the market: cleansing and disinfecting materials, creams, stickers/patches, etc., but not all of these may necessarily be suitable for you. If the preparation you tried didn't help, don't despair. There are other solutions. In general, there should be a real improvement in the condition of your pimples after several weeks. If so, then keep on with the treatment; if not, go to the next stage, and see a dermatologist for more advice.

Some of you may rather see a cosmetician—either before or after going to the pharmacy. The next chapter explains how the cosmetician can contribute to the treatment of acne, but we must stress this right now: If you intend going to a cosmetician, before you entrust her with something so precious to you as your skin, be absolutely certain that she is duly licensed and experienced.

GRADING THE SEVERITY OF ACNE

Mild Acne	Moderate Acne	Severe Acne
Blackheads or whiteheads	Inflamed red pimples, pustules and some cysts.	The whole works: blackheads and whiteheads, inflamed red pimples, pustules and deep cysts. Sometimes also scarring and pigmentation stains.

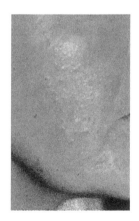 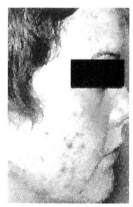 

...Or Dermatologist

Many of you will prefer to go directly to a dermatologist. The physician will diagnose the condition of the pimples, recommend the most appropriate treatment for you, and provide guidance and full medical supervision of the treatment.

It is best to establish a good relationship with the dermatologist based on sincerity and trust. Don't hide from the physician any information that may help with the treatment, even if you are concerned that it is intimate or embarrassing. Keep this in mind: You are not the first to suffer from acne. The dermatologist has already treated hundreds of cases similar to yours. You can rely on his/her experience and discretion.

VISIT TO A DERMATOLOGIST

How to Prepare for the Appointment with the Dermatologist

Some prior understanding may save time and frustration for both you and the doctor. If you are afraid that you may be too stressed and will find it difficult to concentrate, listen or reply, don't be embarrassed to ask a family member or friend to accompany you. Prepare your questions in advance with your parents' help, and assemble beforehand all relevant information (such as similar cases in your family, sensitivity to medications, etc.).

You can expect the dermatologist to ask you preliminary questions such as:

- How long have you been suffering from pimples?
- Are there severe cases of acne in your family?
- What treatments have you already tried (over the counter drugs, cosmetic treatments)?
- Does your acne sometimes get worse when you're under stress, or after using cosmetics, or after eating a particular food?
- Are you sensitive to medications, especially antibiotics, or certain preparations?
- Do you suffer from any illness, or are you taking any medications regularly?
- For women only: Are you suffering from any hormonal disorder? Do your pimples get worse just before you get your period?

Before you leave the doctor's office, make certain that you have the following answers:

- How to use the medication or medications that the doctor prescribes for your treatment.
- How long should it take before there is improvement?
- Can you expect side effects when taking the medication?
- If the treatment fails, what other possibilities are there?

Treatment of acne demands a great deal of patience, decisiveness and self-discipline. These are the essential requirements for anyone who wants to achieve good results in treating this disorder.

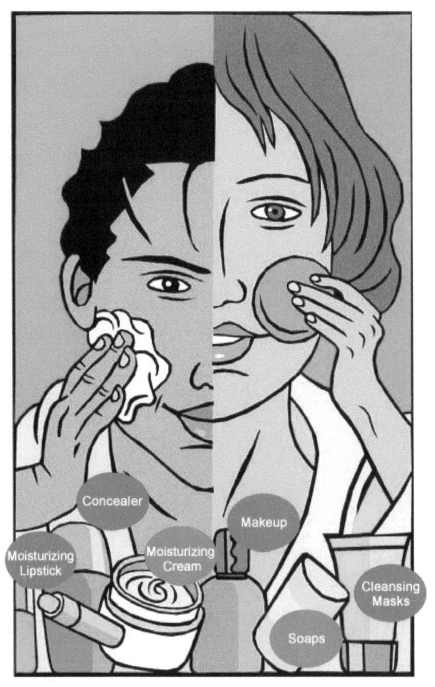

The Acne Solution –

Chapter 5
COSMETIC TREATMENT

Let's go through the everyday activities of cleaning and caring for your skin and possible ways of using makeup to cover pimples. We'll help you find those products that are suited for your skin, and warn you about those that should be avoided. We'll also explain the role of the cosmetician in treating facial skin that is prone to acne.

What Type of Skin is Prone to Acne?

Skin predisposed to acne is defined by dermatologists as oily skin or combination skin. Combination skin is more oily in the center of the face (the notorious "T-zone" as it is called due to its shape, across the forehead, down along the nose and down to the chin) and less oily on the cheeks.

As you may know from your own experience, this definition is much too general. Not everyone with oily or combination skin suffers from acne. On the other hand, there are those whose skin can be defined as normal, perhaps even dry, yet it is not clear of pimples.

Listen Up to a Few Important Comments

Consult your cosmetician in choosing cleansing face-care and makeup preparations. Ask your dermatologist for guidance in integrating these preparations in your medication treatment.

If you are taking medications such as Roaccutane/Accutane for treating acne, avoid using cleansing and care preparations that dry your facial skin. To relieve the sensation of dryness due to the use of certain medications, apply lipstick for dry lips, as well as moisture and sunscreen creams.

All the above information and guidelines for facial skin also hold true for any other areas of your body where pimples may appear.

A Superabundance of Cosmetic Products

The market is flooded with good and suitable cleansing and care preparations, local and imported, making it difficult to choose between them.

CLEANING YOUR FACE

Skin care, even for healthy skin, begins with cleansing. Bacteria multiply more slowly on clean skin and fewer pores become clogged with sebum. When cleansing the skin, we strive to remove dirt, surplus oil and dead skin cells.

At this very moment you are probably thinking, "So what's new about cleaning my face? I've been doing this regularly for years!" Read on, and you may find out that there are some things that you still don't know.

Just Twice a Day. Any More Can be Harmful

Short and proper treatment of facial skin twice a day is the key to keeping your skin healthy. Avoid facial cleansing that is too frequent or too vigorous. It may cause excessive dryness of the skin, redness and itching, and may also aggravate your acne.

What in the Morning? What at Night?

The routine of caring for your face, in the morning and before bed, begins by cleansing the skin with a suitable soap. In the morning, after the cleansing, apply an appropriate moisture cream to your skin, and add a sunscreen lotion before leaving the house. Now, if you want, you can make up your face and conceal the pimples.

Before bedtime it is essential to remove all makeup and the remnants of the care preparations from your skin. If your skin is prone to acne, it is preferable to avoid applying nourishing cream for the night.

Once or twice a week you can use a mask for deeper cleansing of the skin.

PREPARATIONS FOR CLEANSING FACIAL SKIN
Soaps

Soap is a mixture containing sodium or potassium salts of fatty acids with vegetable oil (coconut, palm and others) or animal fat (tallow). Soap manufacturers add to this basic mixture additives such as various minerals or colors and fragrances. Changing the composition of the mixture, and using a variety of additives, results in an abundance of soap types: desiccating (drying) soaps, oily lubricating soaps, perfumed soaps, transparent soaps, colorful and so on. All are intended to remove oil and dirt from the skin.

A mixture of soap and water can penetrate the oily layer enveloping the skin. As this mixture comes into contact with the oil drops and dirt, a chemical process takes place in which they are removed from the skin.

Ordinary soaps do a fairly good job of cleaning the skin, but when cleaning skin with a tendency to acne, they have two disadvantages:

1. They have an alkaline pH and may irritate the skin.

2. Ordinary tap water is "hard," meaning that it contains salt, calcium and magnesium, which tend to combine with the fatty acids in the soap and leave a deposit of insoluble salts on the skin.

You should therefore take care to use a "soapless" soap – a preparation that does not contain sodium or potassium salts. Pick a soap with an acid pH (5-6) similar to the natural acidity of the skin, which does not cause irritation, yet has good cleansing capability.

Avoid scented soaps. Perfume is one of the most common allergens and may irritate the skin. It contributes nothing at all to the efficacy of the soap, but very often raises its price.

The following are a few examples of cleansing materials and soaps that are suited for skin that is prone to acne:

Cleansing Masks

Cleansing masks are applied several times a week and are intended for deeper cleansing of the skin. They act by gently peeling the skin, removing dead cells, and cleaning the pores and blackheads. Masks contain various minerals; and usually skin moisturizing and relaxing substances as well.

The mask, usually a thick mixture, is spread on a clean face and allowed to dry. After a few minutes, according to the instructions on the package, the mask is removed with a moist sponge or with soap and water.

For oily skin we recommend an oil-absorbing mask containing absorptive ingredients. Look for a mask containing clay. Clay, with its exceptional adsorption ability, excels in getting the dirt out of skin pores.

As always, listen to the salesperson's recommendations, but also read the label before buying. Avoid products containing fragrances, as they may irritate your skin.

Here are some examples of masks suitable for skin that is prone to acne:

CARING FOR YOUR FACE

Most likely many of you are very familiar with the following dilemma: Is it better to use care and makeup products to conceal the acne? Or is it preferable to be extra careful and avoid using cosmetic preparations altogether? This conflict is not yours alone. It also preoccupies both the dermatologist and the cosmetician. They are entrusted with the task of recommending preparations that conceal the pimples on your face, but without aggravating the damaged skin. It turns out that this task is not at all simple. Unfortunately, most cosmetic preparations that effectively conceal the signs of acne are oil-based. These may clog skin pores and aggravate the condition.

The physician or cosmetician may not always be able to offer a perfect solution for the unaesthetic blemish that you are trying to hide, but you can depend on them to act responsibly and recommend only products that are safe and fit in with the medications you are already taking.

Which Skin Care Products to Choose...

How can you pick the suitable products out of a vast selection of products on the shelves? There is no exact answer. While there are indeed many such preparations, finding the right ones is a matter of trial-and-error. We recommend first buying the smallest size package (or better yet, get a free sample), so that replacing the preparation by another will not cost you too much money. And just the same: how will you know which preparation to pick and which to avoid?

Here are a few helpful suggestions:
- Consult the dermatologist and cosmetician on choosing the cosmetic product and how to integrate it in your medicinal treatment.
- Don't use a particular product only because your friend uses it. It may not be suitable for you.
- Don't be enticed into buying a preparation manufactured by an unknown company or compounded by a private outfit.
- Buy only oil-free and fragrance-free preparations or those that do not encourage blackheads or whiteheads (non-comedogenic).
- Make sure that you are buying preparations labeled "derma-

tologically tested" or "hypoallergenic." Such labels ensure that these products have been adapted for very sensitive skin.

- When you buy a new product, one that you never used before, try it out for a few days on the inside of your forearm, and apply it to your face only after making certain that you're not sensitive to it.

...And Which Ingredients to Avoid?

Various cleansing and care preparations contain ingredients that may encourage development of blackheads and whiteheads. If you are suffering from acne, or if your skin tends to produce pimples, avoid using these preparations. Avoid: linseed oil, olive oil, sesame oil, peanut oil, cocoa butter, almond oil, coconut oil, oleic acid, butyl stearate, myristoyl, isopropyl, petrolatum, lanolin, mineral oil, bergamot oil, PABA.

SKIN CARE PRODUCTS

Moisturizing Cream

Exposed skin is constantly losing moisture. Water moves by diffusion from deeper layers of the skin to the outer layer where it evaporates. Moistening the skin with water that evaporates freely dries the skin even more because the evaporating water takes with it the moisture of the outer skin layer.

Contrary to what is commonly thought, moisturizing cream does not add water to the skin; it is intended to retain the water already in the skin and prevent its evaporation. So if your skin is short of moisture, the moisturizing cream alone will not improve the condition. Therefore, in addition to the cream, you should drink at least 6-8 glasses of water a day. Avoid staying too long in a room with an air conditioner or heater, as these also dry the skin.

Some soaps and medications for topical (local) use (see the next chapter), such as derivatives of vitamin A and benzoyl peroxide, dry the skin and cause a constant peeling of the outer skin layer. Moisturizing cream soothes the dry and irritated skin and fits in well with the medicinal treatment.

It is very important to choose a suitable moisturizing cream for treating skin with acne:

- A preparation that is oil-free. Oil clogs the openings of the sebaceous glands and encourages the formation of blackheads and whiteheads.
- A preparation that contains sunscreen. If the preparation does not contain this important ingredient, make sure to cover your skin with a cream that protects you against any exposure to the sun.
- Cream containing soothing substances such as aloe vera, pentanol, and herbal essences.
- A cream labeled "dermatologically tested," "for sensitive skin," or "hypoallergenic."
- Moisturizing cream containing alpha hydroxy acids (AHAs). These acids absorb water, promote skin renewal, and clean pores and blackheads.
- Take note: substances such as elastin and collagen are ineffective because their large molecules cannot penetrate the skin.

Examples of moisturizing preparations suitable for acne-prone skin:

Moisturizing Lip Balms

One of the side effects of some acne medications (such as Roaccutane/Accutane, of which you will read extensively in *Chapter 7*) is considerable dryness of the lips. Sometimes the lips also become inflamed, or crack and peel. You can relieve this by using suitable lip balms with high moisturizing ability and containing sunscreen. Look for the label showing it has been dermatologically tested and is hypoallergenic. Since most such lip balms are colorless, they are also suitable for boys and men.

Drying Lotions

This group of products, especially developed for skin with acne, is intended to reduce the amount of sebum secreted by the sebaceous glands and dry the affected skin. The preparations usually also contain disinfecting and soothing ingredients. The lotion is applied to each pimple or a group of pimples, but because of its color and texture, it is usually done before going to bed, for the night only.

Sunscreen Preparations

If you live in a sun-drenched climate, you probably indulge in year-round summer light and warmth, but over the years we learned, some of us the hard way, that sun radiation damage can be serious and irreversible. Today, wiser than ever, we know that we must protect the exposed parts of our body with preparations containing UVA and UVB sunscreens. This applies to all of us at all times (depending on where you live, maybe even in the winter!), particularly to those suffering from acne. There are medications and preparations prescribed for acne that increase the sensitivity of the skin to the sun. Even the lips sometimes become dry and sensitive, and need to be protected.

Skin and face care is incomplete without sunscreen. Adopt a regular habit: Check the ingredients of your care products (such as moisturizing cream or makeup). If they don't contain sunscreen with a rating of 15 at the very least, make sure that your skin is protected with a sunscreen lotion before leaving the house.

Makeup Products

Using makeup requires special attention and much caution. Some preparations may clog skin pores, aggravate the acne, and sometimes even cause an outbreak of the disorder. But you can find skin care and makeup products at the cosmetics counter that are safe to use, even by those with especially sensitive skin and acne sufferers.

Observe a few precautionary rules:
- Use only oil-free preparations.
- Don't apply "heavy" makeup.
- Make certain to remove the makeup every evening before going to bed.
- Use your judgment and use the makeup and skin care products to your advantage.
- Don't let them work against you.

Note: We are mainly referring to foundation preparations intended for basic facial cover. Other makeup products, such as eye shadow, makeup pencils, and lipsticks have no particular effect on acne.

Preparations for Covering Pimples

"If I could only hide the pimples, or at least cover them up." You've probably made this wish quite often. We're sure that if there were a perfect solution for concealing skin blemishes, many people would pursue it no matter the cost.

While unfortunately there is no perfect solution, it is possible, and even recommended, to use special preparations to cover and conceal the blackheads, pimples, and pigmentation stains.

Makeup

A broad variety of foundation preparations await you at the cosmetics counter, including makeup of various textures – powder, liquid, or stick – in a variety of shades, among which you can find the one that suits your skin best.

These preparations are usually intended for girls and women only as part of their makeup routine. But when it comes to hiding pimples, there is no reason why boys can't benefit from the advantage of these products.

In order to be suitable for acne-prone skin, the makeup preparations must be oil-free, water-based and unscented. Just as with the other preparations, make certain that they are hypoallergenic and contain sunscreen.

Cover Stick

A cover stick is used instead of liquid foundation. It is particularly effective when you want to focus on covering a few pimples scattered here and there over your skin, and just conceal them. The stick can also be suitable for everyday use by boys and men for point cover and concealment of pimples and for drying them out.

Makeup Remover

Cleansing your skin before bed includes removing your makeup. You can use special preparations for removing makeup: liquid soapless soap, face milk, face water, or a combination product. Whether you choose these, or go another way, make certain that you are using preparations intended for acne-prone skin.

HAIR CARE PRODUCTS

Preparations designed for caring for your hair, such as shampoo, softener and even coloring preparations, don't really affect acne. As it can be assumed that your hair is oily, since this is a characteristic of acne sufferers, you should use products adapted for oily hair. An exception to this is hair styling gel. As it comes into contact with the skin on the forehead and cheeks, the gel may cause acne. As a rule, you should avoid using oil-based gel, and make certain to first pin up your hair.

Some of you must cope with another annoying esthetic problem: dandruff. It seems that this problem is sometimes caused by a fungus that feeds on the sebum and tends to develop in an oily environment. Fortunately, dandruff can be controlled by using a special shampoo for this purpose. Make sure you use it according to the manufacturer's instructions. We recommend washing your hair often enough to remove the surplus oil.

Products for Men

Today, most of the well-known cosmetics companies offer a special line of products just for men. The lines include all the important skin care preparations such as moisturizing cream, various concealing preparations, and aftershave preparations. The care products for men are "lighter," more delicate in texture and with less scent than those manufactured for women. Other than that, there are no substantial differences between the two product lines. In any case, it is recommended that the males who are reading this also read this chapter from the beginning.

SHAVING AND SHAVING PRODUCTS

Shaving could be a very complicated and traumatic experience for boys and men with acne, particularly when suffering from pustules, but don't give up on it. Shaving is important for cleaning the skin. If shaving skin covered with pimples causes you discomfort, or makes the pimples worse, you can shave less frequently, maybe every other day.

What is Better: Razor Blade or Electric Shaver?

There is no one answer. Some prefer the razor blade, while others think that the shaver is the correct choice. Try one or both and decide which one you personally prefer. In both methods, it is recommended to shave only in the direction in which the hair grows.

Proper Shaving

A few suggestions for proper shaving of skin with acne:
• Before shaving, wash your face with hot water.
• If you prefer an electric shaver, first use a lotion intended to reduce skin irritation.
• If you have chosen to use a razor blade:
• If your face skin is sensitive, try using a special gel for sensitive skin instead of shaving foam.
• Leave the shaving gel, or foam, on the face for a few minutes before beginning to shave.
• Use the new generation flexible razor blades, and change them often.
• Wet the razor blade in cold water and make certain to rinse it frequently during shaving. Rinsing removes shaving materials and soap from the blades.
• To avoid nicking yourself while shaving, don't stretch your skin too tightly.

After Shaving

Since shaving with a razor blade or electric shaver dries and irritates the skin, you should use an aftershave lotion. Avoid using alcohol-based spray that dries the skin.

A few more suggestions for selecting an aftershave preparation:
• Look for a preparation that contains moisturizing ingredients and skin soothing agents.
• Choose a product that also contains sunscreen.
• It would be best to pick a preparation that contains antibacterial or disinfectant substances, in order to prevent skin infections.
• As with any preparation intended for skin with acne, here too, make certain that the label states "dermatologically tested" or "hypoallergenic."

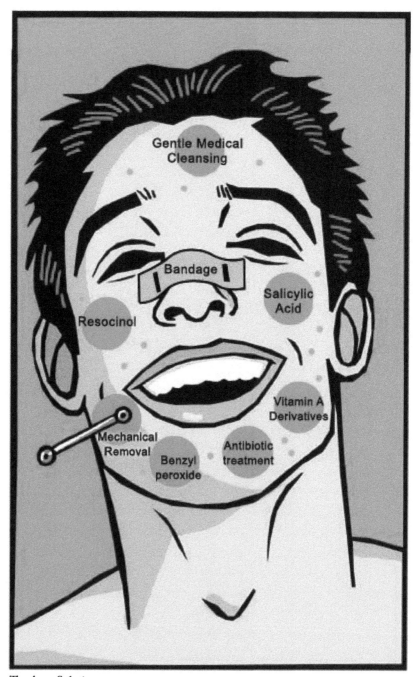

The Acne Solution –

Chapter 6

TOPICAL TREATMENT OF ACNE

Let's now review the products suitable for topical (local) treatment of acne. These are the preparations that are applied to the skin directly at the place where the pimples erupt. Some of these products maintain skin cleanliness, while others are intended to treat pimples of various degrees of severity—from blackheads or whiteheads to reddish papules, with or without pus.

Topical preparations act slowly and require patience and persistence. If the condition shows no improvement within a few weeks or months from beginning treatment, return to the physician and try a different approach.

Some preparations for topical treatment of skin require a doctor's prescription and strict medical supervision throughout the entire course of treatment. If you develop a sensitivity (allergy) to the medication, or should an undesirable side effect appear, stop using it and see your doctor.

SKIN DISINFECTANT PRODUCTS

Medical Disinfectant Products

Available to you is a selection of soaps, lotions and creams containing medical disinfectants (antiseptic) that destroy or block the development of bacteria. The action of these preparations— such as Polydin Soap and Dermex, is stronger than that of the cosmetic cleansing products described in the previous chapter, but they are not widely used, mostly because they dry the skin and can irritate it as well. Today we are inclined to recommend preparations with gentler action, such as Cetaphil, Alpha Clean or Sebamed. While these do not require a prescription, it would be best to consult a pharmacist or a cosmetician before use.

Chemical Antibacterial Products

Sulfur and calamine with sulfur, are chemical antibacterial preparations, acting against the bacteria that causes acne. The ingredients penetrate into the hair follicle, destroy the bacteria, and avert the inflammatory reaction.

What About Side Effects?

Disinfectants may dry and irritate the skin. Using them less often while applying a water-based (reduced oil) moisturizing cream could improve the condition of the skin.

PREPARATIONS FOR DISSOLVING BLACK-HEADS OR WHITEHEADS

Alongside the medical preparations, a number of mechanical means developed in recent years are intended to remove blackheads and whiteheads.

Stickers for Removing Blackheads

These special stickers are moistened and placed on the skin. After a few minutes they are carefully removed, taking with them the blackheads that have been drawn out from the skin pores. Using stickers is easy and fast, and this action can be repeated once or twice a week. It should be kept in mind though that this action does not prevent the appearance of new blackheads.

Also, these methods are not for everyone. Before buying a product, read the manufacturer's instructions on the package carefully and note possible side effects.

Device for Removing Whiteheads and Blackheads

This is a simple, yet effective device for removing whiteheads and blackheads. At one end is a sort of small spoon, perforated in the center. Its other end is sharpened to a point. Piercing the whitehead with the pointed end, placing the spoon over its opening, and pressing with moderate force, will extract it.

When extracting a blackhead, the pointed end is not used. Placing the spoon over the blackhead and pressing moderately does the job.

Treatment is performed by a cosmetician and, in rare instances, a doctor.

Cosmetic Masks

A cosmetic mask helps remove blackheads and whiteheads through very gentle skin peeling. The treatment can be done by a cosmetician, or it's possible to do it yourself, after getting suitable instructions.

Keratin

Keratin, the protein that accumulates in the hair follicle and forms a plug that clogs it, is one of the "culprits" in the formation of acne. The keratin dissolving preparations listed below penetrate the skin pores and help remove dead skin cells, enabling the sebum to drain freely to the skin surface. Drainage prevents accumulation of sebum and the development of non-inflammatory pimples.

Salicylic Acid Preparations

No need for prescription. Consult with pharmacist

Salicylic acid preparations, sold in gel, ointment and liquid form, are intended for treating mild acne. In certain cases, in combination with other substances for topical treatment or taken orally, they are beneficial whatever the severity of the acne. Their application causes the keratin plug to dissolve and reduces skin oiliness. As long as your skin tolerates acid well, you should use it as part of the skin cleansing process.

What about side effects? Since salicylic acid preparations may cause dryness and irritation of the skin, it would be wise to avoid applying other substances that dry the skin at the same time. An oil-free (water-based) moisturizing cream is a very effective means for relieving irritation, and its application enables the skin to adapt to the acid after a week or two.

A few users may develop sensitivity to salicylic acid, and irritation and redness of the skin may occur. If this happens, use of the preparation should be stopped at once. In all events, salicylic acid should not be applied to large areas of the skin.

Resorcinol

No need for prescription. Consult a pharmacist.

Resorcinol is a long-standing medication used for topical treatment of acne. It is intended for mild acne, and in combination with other preparations, for all levels of the disorder. It is useful for opening the keratin plug, and has some antibacterial properties as well.

What about side effects? This substance may cause skin irritation and even a change in hair color and in the color of clothing that comes in contact with it.

Resorcinol should not be used for treating open wounds.

While using the preparation, prolonged exposure to the sun should be avoided.

Vitamin A Derivatives

Prescription Required

Clogging of the hair follicle, a stage in the formation of acne, is caused due to irregular growth of skin cells lining the channel. Vitamin A promotes proper growth of the cells, and helps prevent the formation of the keratin plug.

Vitamin A derivatives act in a controlled daily regimen by lightly peeling the skin, removing the dead skin cells, assisting in eliminating blackheads and whiteheads, and promoting formation of smooth and uniform skin. Vitamin A increases the production of collagen, which serves as the base for the skin's connective tissue. Its action may help in removal and "micro" smoothing of lumpy scar tissue.

As a result, vitamin A derivatives are considered the leading products in topical treatment of acne in its various forms, alone or in combination with other substances.

Vitamin A derivative preparations for topical treatment of acne are sold in cream, gel and solution form.

Directions for using vitamin A derivatives: The directions for use inserted with the preparations should be strictly followed. Here are the principal guidelines:

Thin layer: Apply a very thin layer on clean and totally dry skin, free of makeup or any cosmetic creams whatsoever. Using excessive amounts may cause skin irritation.

Cover the entire area: Apply the medication over the entire area affected by pimples, not only on the pimples themselves. Many clogged hair follicles are so minute that they cannot be seen. It is important to avoid applying it near the eyes or other mucous membranes (nose, mouth).

Increase gradually: Vitamin A derivative products are available with different concentrations of active ingredients. At the outset of treatment, it is recommended, in consultation with your dermatologist, to use a preparation with a low concentration, increasing gradually until reaching the indicated concentration.

After dark: These medications are to be applied only after dark, since exposure to light may reduce the effectiveness of the medication. Exposure to sunlight of skin treated with vitamin A may also increase the skin's sensitivity. Leave the preparation on the skin overnight and wash it off the next morning. Use a sunscreen preparation during the day for protection against the sun, and a moisturizing cream to prevent dryness and inflammation.

How long does treatment last? Although vitamin A preparations do not affect the skin right away, in the course of the first two months you will begin to sense a change in your skin's texture. After continuous use over several months, blackheads and white-heads will disappear, and open pores will close and shrink.

What about side effects? Local irritation of the skin might be caused by using a vitamin A preparation for several reasons: using excessive quantities of the preparation, local sensitivity due to contact with the preparation, and an increase in enlarged blood capillaries, and exposure to the sun which may lead to a burn-like reaction on the treated skin.

At times the skin could turn reddish, dry, or very inflamed, and could start peeling. In such event, the physician may recommend that you switch to a lower concentration of the preparation, or stop using it for a few days and then resume use gradually, or alternately, to allow the skin to adapt.

New vitamin A derivatives (Adaferin, for example) available on the market are less irritating to the skin, do not deteriorate in sunlight, and produce excellent results.

Use of preparations of this group is prohibited for pregnant or nursing women.

TOPICAL (LOCAL) ANTIBIOTICS

For many of us, the term "antibiotics" is related to medications taken orally. However, antibiotic ingredients are also included in preparations intended for topical treatment of inflammatory acne. These preparations are found as lotions, solutions or ointments that penetrate the skin and destroy the bacteria involved in the inflam-matory process. In these forms, the medication reaches the skin directly, at the place it is needed, maintains a high concentration of the active ingredient, and avoids side effects typical of antibiotics that are taken orally.

Erythromycin and clindamycin are most common antibiotic active ingredients in preparations for topical treatment. In addition to these, there are other antibiotic preparations such as Garamycin, Fucidin, Mupirocin, Synthomycin, etc. Each of the antibiotic preparations may be used in combination with other preparations, such as vitamin A. At night, the vitamin A preparation is applied, while the antibiotic is used during the day.

A unique and well-known substance that is very central in treating pimples is benzoyl peroxide. It is dual acting, both as an antibacterial agent and in dissolving the keratin plugs.

The effect of topical antibiotic treatment is not immediate, but after some time (ranging from several weeks to a few months) a real improvement will take place in the condition of the acne, perhaps even leading to complete healing. If treatment is successful, but new pimples appear on your skin some time later, return to the doctor, who will either write you another prescription for the same preparation or recommend a different treatment.

At times, in spite of the topical antibiotic application, new pimples appear in the course of treatment. This happens when some of the bacteria on the skin develop resistance to certain antibiotic drugs. This problem can be overcome, however, by using preparations that combine an antibiotic ingredient with another substance (such as benzoyl peroxide) or by replacing the type of antibiotic.

What About Side Effects? Alcohol, an ingredient in some of the antibiotic solutions, may dry and irritate the skin, but since the skin of most acne sufferers is oily, it easily tolerates these preparations. For sure, if your skin is sensitive, you should avoid using solutions and prefer the antibiotic in lotion or ointment form. If your skin feels dry, oil-free moisturizing cream may provide relief.

Listen up! Some antibiotic preparations are prohibited for use by children, during pregnancy and nursing, and by those who are sensitive to specific drugs. Consult your doctor and study the directions inserted with the preparation carefully.

BENZOYL PEROXIDE

No prescription required – consult the pharmacist

Benzoyl peroxide is used in industry to whiten flour, but we are more interested in its contribution to treating acne by destroying the bacteria that cause inflammatory pimples. Such bacteria develop only in the absence of air; in conditions such as exist in the hair follicle. Benzoyl peroxide, an oxidizing agent, releases oxygen into the follicle, which then destroys the bacteria and helps prevent the formation of new pimples.

Benzoyl peroxide is in the forefront of preparations for topical treatment of all degrees of acne. While its principal contribution is in healing papules and pustules, it also affects blackheads and whiteheads. If your face is covered by many blackheads and white-heads, try using benzoyl peroxide in combination with salicylic acid, or, with the doctor's consent, with vitamin A derivatives. Such and other combinations make the treatment more effective and produce better results.

What about side effects? Benzoyl peroxide may cause skin irritation, so you should use it sparingly. Preparations are available in different concentrations of the active ingredient, ranging from 2.5% to 10%. Start with a low concentration and after a few weeks, when your skin has adjusted to the medication, shift gradually or alternately to a higher concentration. When purchasing the product, consult a pharmacist, who may recommend a product such as Benzac, which contains benzoyl peroxide but is less irri-tating to the skin.

If your skin turns dry, use moisturizing cream. If your skin becomes very red and starts peeling, stop using the product for a few days and then resume using it gradually or alternately.

Listen up! Many beloved blouses, shirts and colorful bedding have been ruined in the course of this treatment. Benzoyl peroxide is an oxidizer and a bleach. It may change the color of fabrics that come in contact with it. Even more, contact with the hair may change its color to an undesirable shade.

In short: **Caution!**

COMBINED PREPARATIONS

Prescription required

Sometimes the doctor prefers to prescribe a specific combination of ingredients rather than rely on the available combined prepara-tions. Be aware that a preparation prepared independently may not always be stable, and its lifetime as an active and effective preparation is limited.

Two types of combined preparations are commonly available:

1. Erythromycin or Clindamycin with benzoyl peroxide
2. Neomycin with Steroid

Benzamycin gel combines benzoyl peroxide with erythromycin. This combination maximizes the advantages of each of the ingredients: opening clogged pores and antibacterial action. The preparation should be kept in a dark and cool place, since it breaks up quickly when exposed to heat and light.

The other preparation is Neo-Medrol, combining neomycin, sulfur, and steroids with antibacterial and anti-inflammatory action.

Due to side effects of the steroids, this preparation should be used with care, and on as small a surface as possible, and for a limited amount of time.

OTHER PREPARATIONS LIST OF TOPICAL TREATMENTS

Azelaic Acid – requires a prescription

In recent years, this acid has been integrated in the topical treatment of mild to moderate acne. Antibacterial, it is also effective for lightening pigmentation stains. Patience is needed though, as the effect of this product becomes noticeable only after a few weeks. Side effects, in the form of slight irritation of the skin to redness and dryness, are rare.

Rozex – requires a prescription

This preparation is based on an antibiotic ingredient, metronidazole, at 0.75% concentration. Available as a gel, it is mostly used for cases of Acne Rosacea, a disorder that affects adults (see *Chapter 10*), and in certain cases for mild to moderate acne.

Always read the leaflet attached to the preparation or medication, even if prescribed by a doctor.

Listen up! Some people may develop sensitivity to a particular medication, and every medication may have various side effects for the individual user.

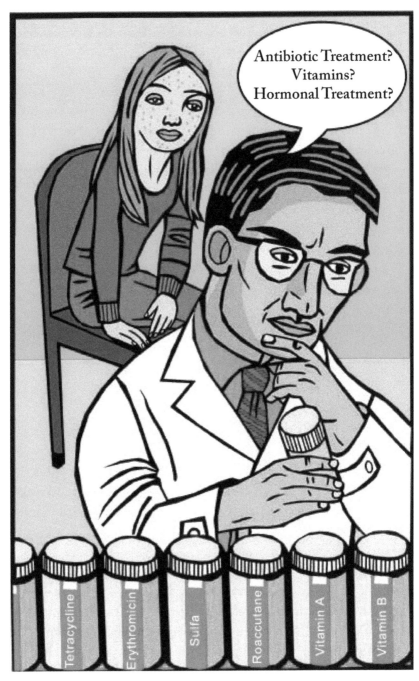

The Acne Solution –

Chapter 7
TREATING ACNE WITH ORAL MEDICATIONS

If your acne is moderate to severe, and does not respond to topical external treatment, your physician may recommend moving to the next stage: oral medications. This type of treatment requires a doctor's prescription and strict medical supervision throughout its entire course.

ANTIBIOTIC TREATMENT

The aim of antibiotic treatment is to heal the infection and inflammation created in the sebaceous glands and the skin. Antibiotics prevent pimples from getting worse and reduce the risks of cysts and scarring.

Antibiotic pills taken orally are absorbed in the blood and enter the skin through the bloodstream. As you continue to take the drug, it gradually accumulates in the skin until reaching a level at which it can eradicate bacteria. Antibiotics have no effect, whatsoever, on blackheads and whiteheads.

Usually, treatment with antibiotics is combined with preparations for topical external use (reviewed in *Chapter 6*). Such combinations improve their efficacy.

Antibiotics – Directions for Use

Antibiotics should be taken only according to a doctor's prescription and directions, in the proper dosage, at indicated times and for the duration required – no matter how long. Observing these guidelines enables the medication to build up to the needed level in the skin which must be maintained throughout the entire course of treatment. If not, it may lead to the development of a strain of bacteria resistant to the drug.

Don't stop the antibiotic treatment on your own before completing it, unless it causes undesirable side effects. If this does happen, you must visit your doctor as soon as you can.

Remember! Only your doctor, who is familiar with your medical background, is qualified to prescribe antibiotics for you. Under no circumstances should you take antibiotics orally on your own or on advice from friends.

How Long Will Treatment Last?

Antibiotic treatment of acne takes a long time. Reaching the required drug level takes about a month. Only then does the healing process begin; and usually lasts at least three months. When the skin is clear of pimples, the doctor will gradually reduce the dosage of the antibiotic until treatment ends. Should pimples reappear, go back to the doctor to resume the treatment, or to try a different treatment.

Can Long-Term Use of Antibiotics Be Harmful to Your Health?

Many believe that antibiotics expose the body to infection by weakening the immune system, but there is no scientific basis for this. Taking antibiotics for treating acne, under medical supervision, when no side effects are produced, will not damage your health, even with prolonged use. A few days after you discontinue the antibiotic, your body will simply "forget" that it has ever consumed it.

What About Side Effects?

Just like any medications, antibiotics have side effects. Most of these are minor and reversible, meaning that they vanish when treatment is stopped. **You should, however, check the known side effects of the medication that you are taking. Talk about it with the doctor and read the leaflet inserted with the medication very carefully.**

On its journey to the skin, the antibiotic may also produce undesired side effects, and even affect other organs of the body. Prolonged use of antibiotics can sometimes cause secondary infections, such as Candida in the digestive system or in the vagina. Should Candida occur, it can be treated effectively while the antibiotic treatment is continued.

Antibiotics and Birth Control Pills

Once it was assumed that birth control pills became less effective while taking antibiotics. In practice, this is very rare. Just the same, **listen up!** If you are beginning to take antibiotics, and you're already on the pill, it would be wise to use additional means of birth control, such as condoms, during the first month of the antibiotic treatment.

If you suspect that you are not properly protected against pregnancy, consult your gynecologist.

OTHER ANTIBIOTIC PREPARATIONS

Your doctor will at first most likely prescribe for you an antibiotic of the tetracycline group. This is the most common antibiotic treatment for acne. If this is unsuitable for you, the doctor has other antibiotics at his disposal.

Tetracycline Group
Drugs of the tetracycline group tackle infection and inflammation in the sebaceous gland, and a distinction is commonly made between first generation and second generation drugs. Since absorption of tetracycline into the bloodstream is affected by the food content in the stomach, they should be taken one hour before or after a meal. Consumption of milk products and products containing iron (and iron preparations) is to be avoided as well, since these impair the absorption of the antibiotic. Due to the rapid breakdown of first generation drugs in the body, they need to be taken 3-4 times a day.

Minocycline and doxycycline are examples of the new generation tetracyclines, and are preferred to the drugs previously used in treating acne. Taken once a day, their absorption into the bloodstream is almost unaffected by mealtimes. Treatment is effective and more convenient compared with the former drugs, but they are more expensive.

What About Side Effects?
As a rule, using drugs of the tetracycline group is safe and there are no restrictions on taking them for lengthy periods. Still, they could have side effects. If you are taking drugs of this group for a prolonged period, the doctor will recommend that you undergo annual checkups for liver and kidney function.

Some of the side effects can definitely be prevented if proper care is taken. You should especially pay attention to the following:

Taking tetracycline, especially together with birth control pills, may increase sensitivity to sunlight. Overexposure to the sun may cause severe sunburn and pigmentation stains, especially on the face. It is therefore highly recommended to avoid tanning and protect the skin with sunscreen.

Tetracycline treatment should not be combined with vitamin A or Roaccutane/Accutane (see below).

Treatment with these drugs is not recommended for children under 12, since prolonged use may harm milk teeth and affect their color.

Drugs of this group are prohibited for pregnant women.

Erythromycin

Erythromycin is used to treat those who cannot be treated with tetracycline, such as children, or pregnant women. These antibiotics, belonging to the macrolide group, are also separated into several generations. Those of the new generation (such as roxithromycin and azithromycin) are more effective and produce fewer side effects than the former drugs.

These drugs have very few side effects, except for nausea and stomachache.

Sulfa

Sulfa is suitable for treating stubborn acne. It often succeeds when other antibiotics fail. Some people develop an allergic reaction to sulfa. It may also increase sensitivity to sun and cause, due to exposure to the sun, harsh skin rashes. Therefore, when taking sulfa, your skin should be well protected by sunscreen. Sulfa is prohibited for anyone suffering from G6PD enzyme deficiency (favism, sensitivity to fava beans), as using the drug may cause the breakdown of red blood cells.

Other Antibiotic Preparations

The antibiotic preparations mentioned here are the most accepted and common, but there are of course others. The doctor may recommend another type that is appropriate for you.

ROACCUTANE/ACCUTANE
(Isotretinoin)

Roaccutane/Accutane is a vitamin A derivative. Its action is similar to that of vitamin A, but much more effective. These products entered the market in 1983 and caused a revolution in the treatment of acne. Stubborn pimples that for years did not respond to other therapies went away after a single course of treatment. These medications produces excellent results, and their use is ever popular.

Who Can Be Treated with Roaccutane/Accutane?

Roaccutane/Accutane is suitable for treating persons suffering from medium to severe forms of acne, and those whose acne — in all forms — does not respond to other medical therapies. The medication is also effective in treating persons with oily skins who suffer from blackheads or whiteheads.

The earlier the stage at which treatment begins the less the risk of developing scars in the affected area.

Roaccutane/Accutane is not recommended for children, but treatment may be started at the age of 12 in severe cases. Adults may be treated with it as well.

How Does it Work?

Roaccutane/Accutane is unique in that it affects the mechanism generating the pimples, as well as the pimples themselves. It works on four parallel tracks:

- Sharply reduces production of sebum, thus preventing clogged pores, the main culprit in the development of acne
- Affects the manner in which skin cells grow. Normal skin cell growth regulates the buildup of the outer skin layers and the inner lining of the hair sheath, thus preventing formation of the keratin plug and clogging of the pores
- Acts indirectly on acne bacteria and reduces skin inflammation
- Alleviates the inflammatory process around acne sores by acting on the immune mechanism

How Successful Is the Treatment?

No other medication is as effective. In 80% of acne cases, complete success is achieved after just one course of treatment. An additional course is required for 15% of the patients, particularly if the first course was not completed, or if the acne (in women) stems from hormonal problems. Five percent of users have to discontinue treatment due to their inability to tolerate the drug or its side effects, or because they fail to respond to the therapy due to unknown reasons.

What About Side Effects?

Taking Roaccutane/Accutane may lead to side effects similar to those caused by an overdose of vitamin C. Fortunately, these side effects are tolerable in most cases, do not require the discontinuation of the medication, and disappear when treatment has ended. Some of the side effects:

- The most common, affecting almost everyone who takes the medication, is dryness of the lips and skin. Suitable ointments and lipsticks are helpful in moistening and lubricating the lips, while moisturizing soap and oily moisture cream may be used to relieve skin dryness.
- Dryness of the mucous membranes of the nose and eyes is sometimes experienced. If you tend to suffer from nosebleeds or wear contact lenses, particularly soft lenses, you must notify your physician, who may then prescribe a lower dosage of the medication.
- Hair may also become dryer, and sometimes hair loss may take place, an occurrence that passes after treatment has ended.
- Taking Roaccutane/Accutane may cause greater sensitivity to sunlight, manifested by redness of the skin. Taking precautionary measures, such as using sun filters and reducing exposure to the sun will enable safe use of the medication during the summer months as well.
- Roaccutane/Accutane may affect the blood fat level. Persons with a genetic disposition to surplus fat in the blood and women on birth control pills are more affected by this. Their blood fat level needs to be tested in the course of treatment. Should

the level rise, the physician may recommend a low-fat diet or prescribe additional medications.

When is Use Prohibited?

Roaccutane/Accutane may cause damage to embryos, **so pregnant women must absolutely not take the drug!** More than that: care must be taken not to become pregnant for one month after completing the treatment with Roaccutane/Accutane.

Roaccutane/Accutane must not be taken if a blood test prior to commencing treatment shows elevated liver function indicator levels.

Should blood tests monitoring liver function show any deviation during Roaccutane/Accutane treatment, the physician may decrease the dosage or stop the treatment completely.

Should unusual headaches develop while taking Roaccutane/Accutane, treatment should be stopped at once and a physician consulted.

Directions for Use

Treatment duration: A course of treatment with Roaccutane/Accutane lasts from four to six months. In many cases the acne may be aggravated in the first month of therapy, but this is a common and predictable response. Gradual improvement takes place in the ensuing months, following which healing will continue at even a faster rate. In most people, the skin is completely cleared of pimples after three to four months, although there are those who do need lengthier therapy.

If you're not as lucky, and your pimples are stubborn, your physician may consider repeating the process and carrying out additional courses of treatment under medical supervision.

Boys who don't respond to Roaccutane/Accutane after several courses of treatment are usually referred for hormone therapy. They may be suffering from a rare hormonal disease of genetic origin, which may erupt during adolescence.

When the basis for acne is hormonal among girls, they may need hormone therapy along with Roaccutane/Accutane, and even afterward.

Treatment continuity: It is undesirable to stop treatment with Roaccutane/Accutane before its completion. However, if for some reason it is discontinued, it can be resumed at a later date under medical supervision.

When is it taken? Roaccutane/Accutane is taken according to physician's instructions, either once or twice a day with a meal, so that it is more easily absorbed by the body. If you miss one or more doses, don't complete what you missed! Just continue taking the regular dosage.

How much? The dosage of Roaccutane/Accutane is determined by body weight. The heavier you are, the larger and more expensive the dosage that the doctor will prescribe. There are those who believe that it is worthwhile losing those extra pounds before beginning treatment!

Dosage ranges from 0.5 mg to 1 mg per kilogram of body weight (and not more than 80 mg per day), and as mentioned, for a period 4 – 6 months on the average.

In certain cases, such as stubborn reappearance of mild forms of acne, or in cases of oily skin that is resistant to treatment (seborrhea), alternate treatment with Roaccutane/Accutane twice a week, one week per month, minimal daily dosage, etc., may be administered for a lengthy period under medical supervision.

What is allowed and what is forbidden? As a rule, taking Roaccutane/Accutane will not change your normal lifestyle.

The medication does not affect the menstrual cycle, does not harm appetite, and does not lead to weight gain or loss. In the course of treatment with Roaccutane/Accutane it is, however, advisable to avoid fatty foods that could increase the blood fat level.

No alcoholic beverages should be consumed while taking Roaccutane/Accutane in order to avoid causing liver damage. Anyone who had hepatitis in the past – but suffered no liver damage – may take Roaccutane/Accutane. Inoculation against hepatitis also doesn't interfere with the treatment, but you should consult with your doctor before being inoculated.

Roaccutane/Accutane may be taken together with birth control pills or with various antibiotics. Exceptions to this are drugs of the tetracycline group. Roaccutane/Accutane should not be taken with drugs from this group.

In the course of treatment with Roaccutane/Accutane, it is also wise to abstain from certain cosmetic procedures. Hair removal with wax may injure the delicate skin, while skin peeling is not recommended due to the risk of scarring. It is also recommended to put off such procedures for some time after completing the Roaccutane/Accutane treatment. In all events, a physician should be consulted.

Summary

Among those who seek treatment for acne, there is some apprehension, although unjustified, about using Roaccutane/Accutane. Roaccutane/Accutane is a most effective medication for treating acne, especially in cases where pimples don't respond to other therapies. In most cases it cures them completely. The medication produces temporary side effects that pass after treatment is completed. Under medical supervision, which is required throughout the entire course of taking Roaccutane/Accutane, there is no reason whatsoever for apprehension about taking the drug. It is just as safe as antibiotics or hormone pills.

Treatment with Accutane/Roaccutane/Accutane eliminates acne effectively and quickly. It also saves exhausting medical therapies and many years of discomfort.

HORMONAL TREATMENTS FOR WOMEN

The purpose of hormonal treatments in women is to reduce the effect of the male hormone testosterone on the skin.

In women, the male hormone originates from two sources: internal – secreted by the ovaries and the adrenal gland —and external—such as beginning or ending the use of birth control. A hormonal imbalance due to a surplus of testosterone may be expressed by a disturbance in the menstrual cycle, excessive hairiness, weight gain or hair loss, as well as an outbreak of acne.

To neutralize the hormonal effect on acne, it is important to identify the source of the surplus male hormone. If you are suffering from hormone-based acne, the doctor may refer you to an endocrinologist (medical specialty dealing with the endocrine gland system).

What is the Suitable Hormonal Treatment?
After the endocrinology examination has been completed, the doctor will be able to propose the most suitable treatment for you.

If your hormonal disorder stems from irregular action of the ovaries, the doctor will probably prescribe treatment with Diane 35, or in certain cases, a different pill, sometimes in combination with Androcur.

If your problem stems from irregularities in the activity of the adrenal gland, the doctor will prescribe other hormonal treatments.

Diane 35 and Androcur Pills
Diane 35 is used primarily as an effective means of birth control. These pills contain an ingredient that blocks the action of testosterone on the skin. These pills also succeed in decreasing sebum production in the skin, thereby preventing the formation of pimples.

Diane 35 pills disrupt the hormonal action leading to the outbreak of acne.

If use of these pills is discontinued before the hormonal problem has been solved, the pimples may reappear, so you must continue taking the pills for some time.

Androcur (or Armocur) is a medication based on the same ingredient as in Diane 35, but Androcur is not used as a birth control pill.

How Long Does Treatment Last?
As mentioned, treatment with pills is lengthy. In the first month of taking the pills, the pimples may even worsen, but only temporarily. Afterwards, some relief will be felt, and within some four months, the skin will be cleared of pimples. Since the dosage of the medication cannot be decreased gradually, the doctor may recommend that you continue to take it for an additional period.

If no improvement at all takes place in the condition of the acne within several months of treatment, a different treatment should be considered.

Use of these drugs is safe, even over a long period. During the pill treatment, you need to be under a gynecologist's supervision and take blood tests to monitor liver function, blood fat level and blood clotting function.

What About Side Effects?

Diane 35, as all birth control pills, may have several side effects, including weight gain or chest congestion. We recommend that you read the medical insert carefully before use.

Treatment with Diane 35 is unsuitable for women suffering from obesity, varicose veins in the legs, or coronary disease.

Other Hormonal Treatments

If the origin of the hormonal disorder that is causing acne is in the adrenal gland and not in the ovaries, the doctor will recommend (depending on the type of disorder) treatment with drugs such as aldospirone (spironolactone), or dexamethasone, medications that reduce the effect of testosterone on the skin.

ANTI-INFLAMMATORY MEDICATIONS, VITAMINS, AND MINERALS

In rare cases, when the antibiotic treatment of acne fails and the inflammatory process needs to be suppressed, treatment with anti-inflammatory medications will probably be recommended.

The leading medication in this group is Dapsone, with cortisone, colchicine, and rifampin used sometimes as well.

Dapsone is prohibited for people suffering from G6PD deficiency (favism, sensitivity to fava beans). Using this medication may induce a breakdown of their red blood cells.

If treatment with one of these medications continues longer than three months, medical supervision is required, with monthly doctor visits and blood tests.

Vitamins and Minerals

Use of vitamins and minerals for treating acne was more common in the past, before the era of antibiotics. Older physicians and many patients – and not only those taking vitamin and mineral additives on a regular daily basis – believe that these additives may have a beneficial effect on the condition of the acne.

Do Vitamins and Minerals Contribute to Healing Acne?

Studies show that only a few are effective in treating acne. Vitamins C and E are considered to have a beneficial effect on the skin, but they were not found to be able to heal acne. On the other hand, vitamin A makes a real contribution in healing the disorder, even when it is severe. Vitamins B3, B6 and zinc are also considered to be effective in treating pimples.

Vitamin A

Much has already been written here about the contribution of vitamin A to the treatment of non-inflammatory acne characterized by blackheads and whiteheads. Many medications and preparations for treating the disorder are based on this essential ingredient.

Treatment with vitamin A at times produces side effects, so taking it requires medical supervision. Since vitamin A is fat-soluble, it can accumulate in the body and in high dosages produce symptoms of poisoning. If you are already taking any medications whatsoever for acne (antibiotics of the tetracycline group or Roaccutane/Accutane), you should consult a doctor about adding vitamin A to the treatment.

Vitamin A is not recommended for children, pregnant women or anyone suffering from hypertension.

In its natural form, vitamin A is found in fatty fish, liver, oil, butter and milk products, and eggs, as well as in vegetables and fruit such as carrots, spinach, green peppers, tomatoes and persimmons.

Vitamin B

Vitamin B-complex causes reduction of sebum production by the active sebaceous glands, which is thought to be their contribution to the treatment of acne.

Using birth control pills, drinking alcohol, taking antibiotics (sulfa, for example) for long periods, may slow the absorption of vitamin B in the body. If you require supplementary vitamin B, it would be best to take B-Complex tablets that include all its components (B3, B6, and others).

Vitamin B of all types is water-soluble. This means that there is no risk whatsoever of an overdose, as any surplus quantity will be eliminated in the urine.

Foods rich in vitamin B include egg yolks, milk, meat and fish, cereals and wheat germ, as well as fruit and vegetables such as cabbage, bananas, and avocados.

Mineral: Zinc

Zinc affects the skin and hair. It has anti-inflammatory properties, a positive effect on healing wounds and improving the response of the immune system, as well as a certain effect on weakening the male hormone. These properties can contribute to treatment of acne.

Taking zinc pills may cause nausea. Since an overdose of zinc may cause poisoning, unsupervised and prolonged use of zinc should be avoided.

Zinc can be taken in combination with vitamin B and vitamin A.

Zinc-rich foods include wheat germ, bran, calf liver, beef liver, eggs, peanuts and lentils.

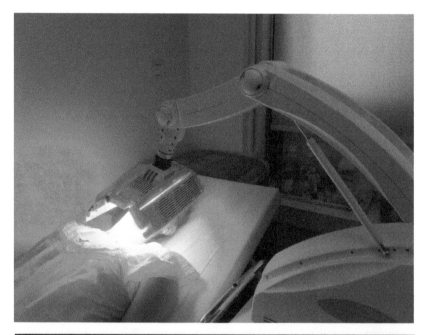

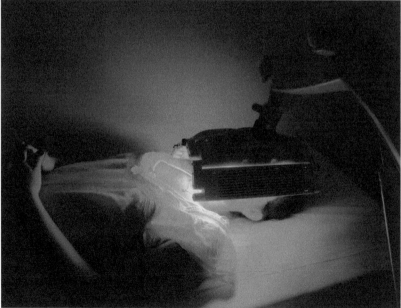

The Acne Solution –

Chapter 8
PHOTOTHERAPHY FOR ACNE: CAN WE TREAT ACNE WITHOUT MEDICATION?

HOW EFFECTIVE IS PHOTOTHERAPY FOR ACNE?

Phototherapy for acne is the fastest treatment available for acne-prone skin. Multi-center studies in five continents have shown that its CureLight's pure violet/blue light effectively clears over 70% of inflammatory skin pimples in just a month. This is just one-third the time of the other traditional acne treatment methods, such as topical creams antibiotics and Roaccutane/Accutane that only start working after four weeks or more of intensive therapy.

Effectiveness of the Light Spectrum in the Selective Destruction of P. Acnes Bacteria and Treatment of Acne-prone Skin

Phototherapy for acne uses the violet/blue part of the spectrum and is UV free. The original Blue Light treatment system developed by CureLight allows much higher power than the common LED light system and is UV free. In contrast to the common LED blue light that emits only blue light, the CureLight system emits, in addition to high intensity blue light, some red and infrared light that have strong anti-inflammatory effects.

Phototherapy Side Effects

Phototherapy for acne is among the safest skin treatments available. Its Selective Photo Clearing technology uses light that is UV free and safe. With phototherapy, there are no known side effects.

Phototherapy for acne can avoid the variety of side effects such as those created by prolonged use of antibiotics or other oral therapies.

Who Can Get Phototherapy? Almost anyone. Phototherapy has been proven to be effective on mild to moderate acne-prone skin. Pregnant women and women who are breastfeeding should consult their physician.

Are Creams Used at Home?

Yes. The skin is thoroughly cleansed with soap prior to treatment sessions and your esthetician will provide you with a lotion such as Glycolic Acid or Benzyl Peroxide for daily maintenance.

How Does Phototherapy Work?

Phototherapy's unique Selective Photo Clearing technology destroys P. acnes bacteria within the skin; P. acnes bacteria are highly sensitive to specific violet/blue light. The UV free light is safe, effective and doesn't cause harm to surrounding tissue.

Does It Hurt?

With Phototherapy for acne a typical treatment session takes only 30 minutes. You sit or lie comfortably while the light is applied. The treatment is very relaxing. Most important: It is painless and safe. Patients often listen to music while being treated.

How Many Treatments Are Required?

Treatments typically involve a series of ten to fifteen sessions performed twice a week. Improvement is typically observed after the eighth session. It is important to keep the treatment appointments recommended by your esthetician in order to hit the P. acnes bacteria at their peak of light sensitivity. By following the treatment plan, you will maximize efficacy and enjoy clearer skin with Phototherapy.

PHOTOTHERAPY BENEFITS

1. Faster results within one month
2. No side effects, painless procedure
3. No downtime – after treatment you immediately return to your daily routine
4. No exposure to antibiotics or other medications
5. Suitable for all body areas, including the sensitive beard, and large areas such as back and chest
6. Avoids the use of risky and less effective lasers or intense pulse-light device.

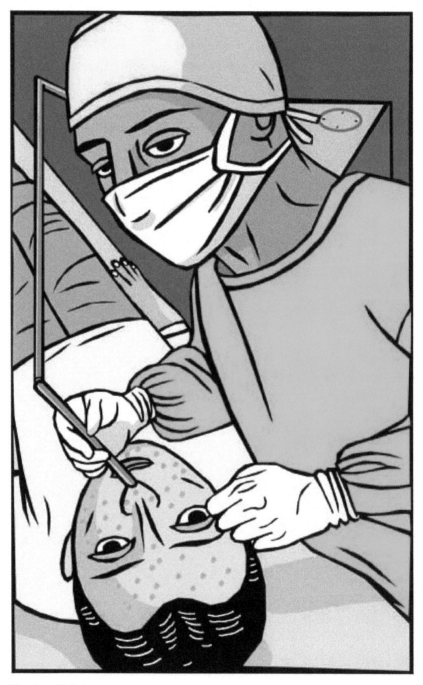

The Acne Solution –

Chapter 9
HOW TO IMPROVE ACNE SCARS WITHOUT SURGERY

There are a few types of acne scars. Some of them are large and shallow (depressed acne scars) and some of them are narrow and deep (ice pick scars). All these scars are hard to treat. The only effective treatments used by doctors in the past were dermabrasion (wire brush "sanding" of the skin), deep laser or chemical peels and microsurgery. As these treatments are frequently associated with prolonged downtime, discomfort, and/or pain, their use decreased.

A new treatment developed in the last few years seems to allow an effective treatment with minimal pain and downtime for the patient. This treatment called "multisource fractional radiofrequency" allows both treatment of the upper surface of the skin (epidermis) to smooth the skin and remove brown spots together with effective deep heating of the dermis to cause production of new collagen that will fill the depressed scar.

WHAT IS FRACTIONAL RADIOFREQUENCY?

The concept of fractional skin resurfacing by laser devices was developed to contend with the shortcomings of ablative and non-ablative device modalities. With these systems, small microscopic "dots" of skin are ablated, allowing for rapid healing with minimal pain and downtime. Although fractional ablation of the epidermis can be achieved with multiple laser systems, the actual dermal volume that is heated by fractional lasers is a very small percentage (5 % - 7 %) of volume. Another problem with lasers is that their penetration to the deep layers of the skin is very low, and they are problematic when used on dark-skinned patients (due to a risk of dark and white skin spots after treatment).

Radiofrequency is the same energy that is used to transmit radio signals. It has been used in medicine very safely for many decades. Radiofrequency has two important advantages over laser treatments. First, it penetrates much better to the deep layers of the skin (dermis) to trigger production of new collagen, and second it is suitable to treat safely all skin types including fair skin and dark skin patients.

WHAT IS THE NEW 3DEEP™ FRACTIONAL RADIOFREQUENCY TREATMENT?

The EndyMed PRO™ System is an FDA cleared computerized system that generates pulses of *radio frequency* (RF) energy directly into the skin. The unique advantage of the EndyMed PRO is that it uses at least six independent sources of RF, instead of the one source used in the other RF systems on the market (Monopolar, Bipolar, "Multipolar"). The uses of multiple sources of RF in the EndyMed PRO allows for both deep dermal non-ablative skin tightening and micro ablative fractional RF skin resurfacing, all on the same system console. With the EndyMed PROs' non-ablative deep dermal hand piece, the dermis can be heated to 55 – 60 degrees Celsius to a depth of up to 11 mm, depending on the hand piece used. The EndyMed Fractional Resurfacing hand piece forms a matrix of 112 tiny RF electrodes, creating small zones of epidermal coagulation with simultaneous volumetric dermal heating of up to 2.8 mm.

WHAT ARE THE ADVANTAGES OF 3DEEP RF TREATMENT OVER OTHER LASERS?

First generation RF systems have one RF generator. The 3DEEP RF technology (EndyMed PRO/Glow by EndyMed) is the only RF system in the world that is based on six independent RF generators allowing a significantly more effective treatment without pain.

This allows fractional surface resurfacing with the high-end lasers providing much more deep heat than other lasers. These specific qualities put the EndyMed system in the top clinics in world, positing the technology as a gold standard both for treatment of acne scars and skin tightening.

WHAT IS EXPECTED DURING THE TREATMENT?

After the treatment area is cleansed the doctor will apply to your skin a topical anesthetic cream to numb the area. After 30 minutes the treatment will be performed. The pain during treatment is very minimal if any. After the treatment, the treated skin will be red for a few hours. On the second day of treatment, small micro crusts were form on the skin, which last up to five days. Multiple studies using this system showed there were no incidences of infection, scarring, hypopigmentation, or any other serious complications in any of the patients.

A recent peer-review published study examined the effects of the combined ablative and non-ablative EndyMed PRO treatment protocol in multiple clinics. The authors concluded that the 3DEEP treatment has shown high patient acceptance with significant clinical efficacy. The non-ablative multisource RF treatment was proved to be painless, while the micro fractional RF skin resurfacing procedure was associated with minimum pain (treatment protocol including the use of a topical anesthetic cream). Since fractional resurfacing with radiofrequency technology results in dry micro ablation, downtime is significantly shorter and the risk for side effects, such as infection, is minimal, as compared to the previous traditional methods of laser resurfacing that result in open wounds, oozing and even bleeding. Clinically, the affected areas are erythematous and mildly edematous after treatment, but this is typically resolved within a few hours. This rapid healing is likely to be related to the persistence of healthy unaffected tissue that remains between the ablated pulses after ablative fractional resurfacing. The incidences of complications and downtime were much lower than in those seen after traditional ablative resurfacing or fractional CO_2 skin resurfacing.

The authors concluded that the new combined protocol, as allowed by the EndyMed PRO, seems to be one of the best solutions for a very effective, minimally invasive, low downtime treatment of depressed acne and traumatic scars.

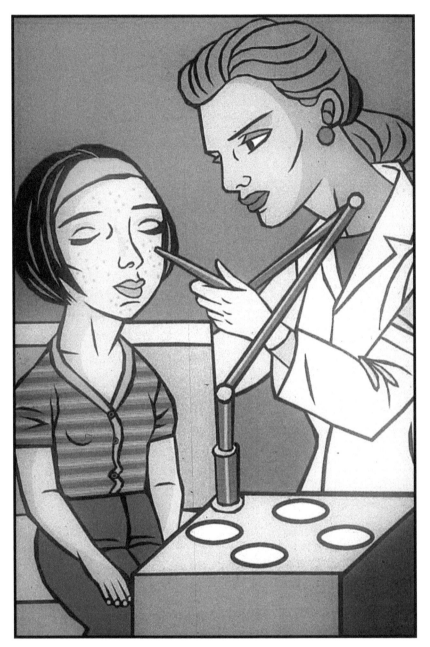

The Acne Solution –

Chapter 10

TREATING SCARS AND PIGMENTATION

Scars, and irreversible marks on the skin, is one of the harshest and most painful side effects of inflammatory acne. Regretfully, scars cannot be completely erased. However, as we will see, by employing certain methods, it is quite possible to minimize their appearance. Scar-filler substances are divided into two categories: permanent and temporary. It is important to understand that the definition is related to the existence of the filler or its reaction on the skin, and not to the actual influence of the active substance. Note that the effective influence of permanent filler might be time-limited. The qualities of ideal filler are: Safety in use, not over sensitivity reaction, not causing infections, easy to store and of course relatively inexpensive. Such an ideal substance is yet to be found. The filler substances listed below are some examples from the approved used substances in different countries.

HOW SCARS ARE FORMED

Scar formation begins with a severe inflammation of the sebaceous gland and the hair follicle. When connective skin tissue involved in the healing process thickens, a raised scar is created in that area. The shrinking of new connective tissue, which causes the skin surface to be drawn inward, forms a sunken scar.

The nature of the scar is affected by its depth, volume and the initial treatment applied. The chances of its healing depend on the individual biological and genetic characteristics of each person.

Some of the crater-like scars improve in appearance with time. At first they are somewhat sunken and reddish. After a few months they become flatter, and their color begins to fade until it blends

How to Identify Your Scar Type

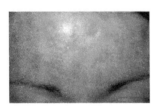

Puncture-Like Scar: relatively deep icepick-like divots.

Sunken Scar: Crater-like scars, concave, rounded, relatively shallow, and sometimes with raised edges.

Keloid Scar: Puffy, raised, and extending beyond the affected area.

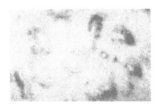

Raised Scars: Hypertrophic **Scar:** Puffy

with the color of the surrounding skin. In such cases, minimum corrective esthetic treatment is required.

The appearance of a scar, whether sunken or raised, is emphasized even more by a factor called the "illumination effect." This effect is produced by the shadow cast on the skin by the light shining on it. When skin is completely smooth, light is scattered uniformly over its entire surface. When light shines on a scar at a non-perpendicular angle, the shadow that forms highlights the skin blemishes. The smoother the scar, the less pronounced the illumination effect, so if the scar on your skin is sunken, suitable treatment will be aimed at filling in the crater with a filler material, or at peeling the scar margins until the appearance of the crater is blurred.

If your scar is raised, the doctor may recommend one of the treatment approaches outlined below, which are aimed at flattening the surface of the scar.

TREATING DEPRESSED SCARS

Filler Materials
Filling sunken scars is performed by injecting filler materials into the dermis layer, under the bottom of the scar. Filler materials increase skin volume, and push the bottom of the scar upward until it aligns with its surroundings, and achieves a flatter appearance.

Temporary filler materials: The effect of biological filler materials is temporary, since they are identified by body's immune system as foreign, which then acts to dissolve and remove them. At times subcutaneous stiffening occurs to form a permanent filler, and improves the appearance of the scar. Injection of biological substances involves minor local pain, but does not usually require any anesthesia whatsoever.

Filler materials based on hyaluronic acid (Surgiderm, Juvederm, Restylane, etc.): Hyaluronic acid, which occurs naturally in the dermis, has a key function in building the skin structure and serves as a base for collagen (Evolance, etc.) and elastin fibers.

Collagen: Collagen was one of the most commonly used materials for filling scars and repairing esthetic blemishes. This protein occurs naturally in the connecting tissue and other tissues.

At first the collagen was taken from dermis layer of cattle, thus forcing doctors to take sensitivity tests before treatment. Despite its safety, the disadvantages of collagen are its short time-span until absorption, and the disappearance of its effect.

About five years ago a new filler was developed by an Israeli company .The development was based on a new technology which resulted in lengthening the effect of the injected filler material and does not necessitate preliminary sensitivity tests. The material is found in various viscosity (density) levels, enabling good flexibility treatments.

Radiesse: This filler is manufactured from a natural substance which is found in bone and cartilage, but not indigenously in the skin. The advantage being its considerable influence even in relatively long period of time (up to 2 years).

Fat: The use of fat tissue is very tempting and promising, since it is taken from the patient's own body, easily accessible, no complication caused by synthetic implants of foreign bodies.

Fat taken from the patient's own body, usually from the derriere, is the safest material for injection. It is not foreign to the body, and so does not trigger undesirable reactions in the skin.

As filler material, fat is suitable for both pit-like scars and crater-like scars.

Since in most cases the blood supply to the fat implants is irregular, they are absorbed by the body and disappear within six months to a year. There are no contraindications to repeating the fat injection process again and again.

Lately (as a result of numerous researches) a new method is being applied: injecting fat, enriched with stem cells, thus optimizing both better absorption of the implant as well as a long-term influence.

The above filler material has become very popular during recent years, because of its effectiveness, and minimum of side effects.

Most products of this group appear in a number of density/viscosity levels, thus enabling maximal compatibility in treatment. Materials of denser levels are used for sunken scars.

Permanent Filler Materials

This group includes synthetic or semi-synthetic materials, or a combination of both. Unlike biological substances, where injection causes swelling and redness and beneficial effects are seen only after several days, non-biological materials improve the appearance of the scars at once. Also, unlike biological materials that eventually are absorbed by the body, the effect of the non-biological materials is permanent.

Artecoll: Artecoll is a combination of a biological material, collagen, with a synthetic material in the form of tiny microspheres. As in any collagen injection, here too a preliminary sensitivity test is required.

Injection of Artecoll is more difficult than collagen injection and requires greater skill from the doctor.

After injection, the collagen is gradually absorbed by the body, while the microspheres remain permanently in the skin and connecting tissue forms around them. Unskilled treatment may cause various and prolonged side effects, such as the formation of small lumps in the skin and a sensation of granularity.

Liquid Silicone: Silicone is a very common synthetic material useful in all branches of industry throughout the world. It appeared on the medical scene in 1930, and has since been increasingly used in the manufacture of disposable medical supplies, prosthetics, implants, etc.

Injections of silicone under the scar cause a predictable moderate inflammatory reaction at the site. Afterwards, some of the stiffness retained by the tissue contributes to the required filling and disappearance of the depressed scar. Silicone is not absorbed by the body, and remains within it permanently.

The problem of using silicone lies in a number of unwanted side effects: over correction due to injecting an overdose of the substance and unforeseen hypersensitive reaction, such as the appearance of lumps called granulomas. This side effect though rare, can also appear many years after treatment. Injection of the substance is debatable and prohibited in most Western countries.

Bio-Alcamid™: This material is combined of a synthetic component (polyalkylamide) and 98% water. Due to the high content of water, the process of injection is accompanied by a great degree of inconvenience and thus requires use of local anesthetics.

The substance reacts as a permanent implant. With time, a capsule is produced around the implant enabling its complete extraction from the skin should the necessity arise. Occasionally, the substance incurs inflammatory and infected reactions.

Aquamid®: A synthetic substance resembling the Bio-Alcamid, but does not arouse the creation of capsules around it. Therefore, it is impossible to extract from skin tissue. Same side effects as Bio-Alcamid.

Sculptra®: Polylactic acid acts as a mechanism of stimulation and local genesis of collagen. Its main aim is to fill volume of the hypodermis. With repeated injections of this substance, one can cause the effect of face lift. Injection of Sculptra can form hypodermis lumps.

SKIN PEELING

The appearance of scars can also be improved by means of skin peeling. The various methods of peeling remove the outer skin layers in order to lower the scar margins to skin surface level.

To preserve the results of the treatment and to prevent pigmentation stains, the doctor will frequently recommend continuing treatment at home through the application of various substances. In addition, anyone who has undergone skin peeling must take care to use sunscreen regularly.

Chemical Peeling

Chemical peeling of the skin utilizing the reaction of the skin proteins to various concentrations of acids causes peeling of the epidermis and part of the dermis, stimulating growth of renewed and healthier skin. The higher the acid concentration, the deeper the peeling achieved and the more blemishes corrected. The length of time the acid remains in contact with the skin may sometimes also affect the depth of the peeling.

Very Superficial Skin Peel

Very superficial skin peel does not lessen acne scars, even though it does have an effect on shallow skin blemishes. Its principal aims are to remove surplus dead cells, unclog skin pores and open blackheads and whiteheads. Very shallow peeling is performed on a daily basis as part of routine skin care.

Suitable active substances for gentle skin peel are vitamin A derivatives (such as Retin-A for external use) in various concentrations (prescription required), and the fruit acid group (alpha hydroxy acids (AHAs)), prominent among which is glycolic acid, produced from sugar cane. Glycolic acid is offered at different concentrations: below 8%, it is considered a cosmetic preparation and no prescription is required.

Superficial Skin Peel

Superficial skin peeling is also not the proper treatment for eliminating scars, but at times it succeeds in improving the appearance of very shallow scars. It is helpful in treating active acne, distended skin pores and pigmentation stains (and also, even though these aren't our concern, in treating tiny wrinkles, sun spots and precancerous spots). To obtain the desired results, several consecutive treatments are needed.

These are carried out by a homogeneous application to the face of glycolic acid in concentrations between 20-70 percent. A cosmetician does lower concentration treatments and a dermatologist does higher concentrations.

A new peeling method, dubbed the "weekend peel," ensures healing of the skin within a few days, enabling rapid return to normal routine. The method is based on combining two peeling techniques: dissolving skin layers with Jessner's solution, and mechanical peeling by using sea coral powder. The combination of these two methods enhances the effectiveness of the treatment and reduces side effects.

Medium-Depth Peel

A medium-depth peel helps to improve the appearance of shallow scars.

This method has many known advantages in treating aging skin, sun and age spots, precancerous skin conditions, etc.

What is the peeling process? A medium-depth skin peel is usually based on using TCA (trichloroacetic acid) of 25 % to 50 % strength.

Preparation for skin peeling involves pre-treatment with other substances, such as Retin-A, Jessner's solution or glycolic acid. The pre-treatment stage helps remove oily deposits from the skin so that during the treatment itself, the acid penetrates deeper into the skin and in a more uniform manner, making the peeling more effective. This stage is not always essential, and it is performed at the doctor's discretion.

During the peeling itself, the doctor uniformly applies acid to the face. The skin begins to peel some four days after application, and continues for seven to eight days.

At the beginning of the process the skin is reddish with some light to medium swelling that eventually recedes. At the end of the peeling process skin color is still reddish-pinkish but lightens, and within another few weeks regains the color of healthy skin.

From this stage onward, use of Retin-A should be resumed on a daily basis. Sunscreen lotions with a high protection coefficient must be used and exposure to sunlight should be avoided as much as possible.

Are there risks and complications? TCA is not toxic and there is no reason to be concerned about any possible internal body injury. Anyone whose skin is dark, however, should avoid using TCA out of concern that pigmentation stains may appear.

The risks in this method are low, although there have been cases of herpes viral infection, bacterial infection, and even scarring, but even if these should occur, all are treatable.

Deep Skin Peel

This treatment provides the maximum benefit possible in flattening crater-like scars.

The method is also used for removing wrinkles and stretching aging skin. The depth to which the solution penetrates affects new and increased production of fibers in the dermis, causing the skin to stretch, and wrinkles to disappear.

What is the peeling procedure? Treatment is under total anesthesia and close medical supervision.

Deep skin peeling is usually done with a phenol solution (carbolic acid) mixed with enteric oils and soap. Two preparations are commonly used: the former, known as the "Baker-Gordon formula," and the newer (developed in Israel), known as the "Exoderm Method." In this method, the epidermis layer is completely liquefied together with the outer and middle layer of the dermis.

After applying the mixture, the doctor covers the patient's face with a sealing mask that helps "liquefy" the skin for a period of 24 hours. In the following days, the skin is treated with topical preparations, such as antiseptic powders, antibiotic creams and Vaseline.

Sometimes, the attending physician also treats the scarred area with mechanical dermabrasion (see below) to deepen the peeling.

The healing process lasts about eight days, after which new, reddish and slightly swollen skin appears. The redness decreases over a period of two months on the average.

Immediately after the face is healed and there is new skin growth, makeup can be applied and matched with the color of the neck area.

What About Risks and Complications?

In dark skin there is risk of pigmentation stains after treatment, so, in cases of severe acne scarring, when deep peel is the only suitable treatment for a dark-skinned person, the doctor may apply anti-pigmentation preparations prior to the treatment. After healing from the peel, these preparations should be used daily over a lengthy period.

If the peel is performed by a skilled doctor, the risks involved in this method are very small, even though there could be bacterial infections and undesirable scarring – all of which can usually be controlled and treated quickly and effectively.

LASER PEELING

Another way of deep peeling the skin is with a very accurate computerized laser device that permits uniform peeling of the skin.

There are two basic approaches to laser peeling: the old one based on ablative laser (co2 or erbium) which resurfacing the skin layers with complete control on the ray penetration and degree of peeling. The new approach is the non-ablative laser treatment that operates on wavelengths that skip over the epidermis layer and penetrate directly into the dermis.

Sometimes a combination of both techniques achieves the perfect results.

What Is the Peeling Procedure?

Peeling is performed under brief and light anesthesia on an outpatient basis (not requiring hospitalization) in an operating room. Afterwards, during the healing period, the skin is treated with Vaseline and cold compresses. After some 10 days, a new cover of reddish and swollen skin is formed. The redness gradually decreases, and within a number of weeks (up to two months), the skin resumes its natural color, although it is sometimes a shade lighter.

Makeup may be then applied to the skin to make it appear tanned, or so that it conforms to the other parts of the neck and upper chest.

What About Risks and Complications?

Possible complications are similar to those of deep chemical peels.

MECHANICAL DERMABRASION

A partial-to-complete solution for crater-like scars and pit-like scars is provided by mechanical abrasion of the skin (dermabrasion). This process is carried out with medical abrasion tools, ranging from sandpaper and machines with crystal burrs to electric high-speed sanding machines. Duration of treatment is about an hour, and it is performed in a sterile environment in an operating room, with local or general anesthesia. Recovery time is eight days to two weeks.

This method is sometimes combined with chemical peel, when it is then possible to deepen the peeling in the scar area and achieve better results. The results of the procedure are usually permanent.

This treatment requires considerable skill on the part of the attending physician, who must manually control the depth of penetration and the peeling process.

What About Risks and Complications?
The mechanical dermabrasion method involves risks of too deep penetration, the formation of secondary scarring, and change in skin color (primarily in dark-skinned people).

RADIO FREQUENCY PEELING
A device was recently developed for controlled skin peeling, employing high frequency radio wave technology. This device enables step by step, layer by layer, planning of the peeling procedure. It is suitable for both superficial and deep peeling, as well as for hiding scars, pigmentation stains, various skin blemishes and wrinkles. The results of treatment by this method have been good, but there is limited experience with it.

TREATING RAISED SCARS
Injecting Steroids
One of the common treatments for shrinking and flattening raised scars (keloid or hypertrophic), is through steroids (cortisone) injection directly into the scar. The best results are obtained when the scar is treated at the very outset, when it is just forming.

Steroids are injected in cycles, once every few weeks, usually without side effects. The injection process involves light local pain in the injection area. At times, several treatment cycles are required, and treatment results are not always satisfactory.

Silicon Gel
Attaching flexible silicon wafers or application of silicone gel for a few months to raised scars throughout the day leads in some cases to flattening.

Apparently, according to theoretical knowledge, the effect of silicon wafers on scars is achieved through the static electricity they produce on the skin surface.

Liquid Nitrogen

Deep freezing with liquid nitrogen (-196Co) sometimes helps flatten raised scars. Treatment is carried out repeatedly once every several weeks by applying the liquid nitrogen to the scar.

Flash Lamp-Pumped Pulsed Dye Laser

Treatment with a flash lamp-pumped pulsed dye laser may be helpful in reducing the volume of raised scars and their typical redness. Treatment is given cyclically, once every few weeks.

The laser beam is released in extremely short microsecond pulses of tremendous force. It is absorbed by oxidized hemoglobin in scar blood vessels, and shrinks the scar by diminishing its blood supply.

Surgical Procedure

Removing a raised scar by surgical procedure necessitates its excision, suturing the area and strict supervision of the wound's healing process. Such surgery is uncommon, since in many cases, a new scar is formed in place of the one that is removed, and sometimes surgery aggravates the condition of the scar.

On the other hand, surgical treatment of cysts is more accepted and effective. The surgeon drains the cyst to permit better access of medication treatment and to prevent deep scarring.

Another surgical technique is intended to repair crater-like scars. The surgeon introduces an ordinary hypodermic needle below the scar and tears the fibers of the thickened connecting tissue. Tearing the fibers frees the bottom of the scar, which then rises to the skin's surface. In most cases, the scar tends to revert to its former condition after some time.

Pigmentation

Pigmentation stains, dark brown stains that appear mostly on the face and sometimes on the back as well, are yet another occurrence that sometimes accompanies inflammatory acne. In a few cases

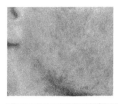 **Reddish-brown pigmentation**

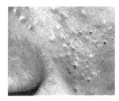 **Inflammatory acne with skin pigmentation**

these are spread over broad areas of skin, while in others they are distributed only as points. Pigmentation stains may remain on the skin for a long time after the pimples have healed.

What are the risks? Let's recap: Picking at acne blemishes increases the risk of inflammation that leaves pigmentation stains. Exposure to the sun encourages the development of melanin cells and the appearance of skin stains. Using birth control pills, or medications of the tetracycline group, also increases the risk of pigmentation, especially if accompanied by exposure to sunlight.

Hormonal disturbances, inclination to anemia due to iron deficiency and various other disorders can also increase the tendency toward pigmentation.

Risk of pigmentation stains is higher among people with dark skin.

Staying Smart—Prevention

The most effective way of fighting pigmentation stains is by preventing them. Visit your doctor early to obtain appropriate treatment of acne, avoid picking and bursting pimples, and avoid violent scraping of facial skin. If you are taking any medication, particularly of the tetracycline group, or birth control pills, inform the doctor and ask the doctor's advice on how to proceed. Reduce exposure to sunlight and be sure to use sunscreen appropriate for your skin type.

Listen up! Pigmentation stains tend to recur. If you fail to strictly practice prevention, then even the treatment that succeeded in removing the stains will not be able to prevent their recurrence. Sticking to the above rules will reduce their recurrence.

Possible to Lighten

If dark stains nonetheless remain on your face, don't despair! There are other ways of lightening stains until the original skin color is restored.

Successful treatment of pigmentation stains naturally depends on the type of treatment, but it also depends on the depth of the pigment in the skin: the shallower the pigmentation, the greater the chance of removal. Dermatologists can determine depth of pigmentation by illuminating the skin stain with a particular wavelength of light from a special lamp.

By yourself or by a Cosmetician

Treatment of shallow pigmentation can be done on your own, or by a cosmetician.

Various fruit, lemons, oranges and strawberries, for example, are known to lighten mild pigmentation stains when applied to the skin. In any case, before starting treatment, consult a cosmetician or a dermatologist.

Many medical and cosmetic preparations for lightening skin stains are available in drugstores, some not requiring a prescription. The pharmacist, cosmetician or dermatologist will help you find the suitable preparation from among the many preparations on the market.

Even if you have opted for treatment by a cosmetician, it is possible that after one or more treatments, you will be able to continue treatment at home, by yourself.

If none of this helps… The dermatologist will select a treatment from among the many treatments available, according to your skin type and pigmentation level.

In mild cases, the doctor usually first proposes a topical treatment preparation such as Retinol, vitamin A (Retin-A), hydroquinone, a special ointment known as the Kligman formula (a combination of hydroquinone and various substances) and azelaic acid.

For more severe cases, the doctor has other solutions such as the daily application of preparations based on fruit acid and other peeling agents, superficial or deep skin peeling, and even treatment with a special laser to lighten the stains.

The doctor will discuss with you the advantages of each treatment and its side effects and will recommend the most suitable treatment for your skin.

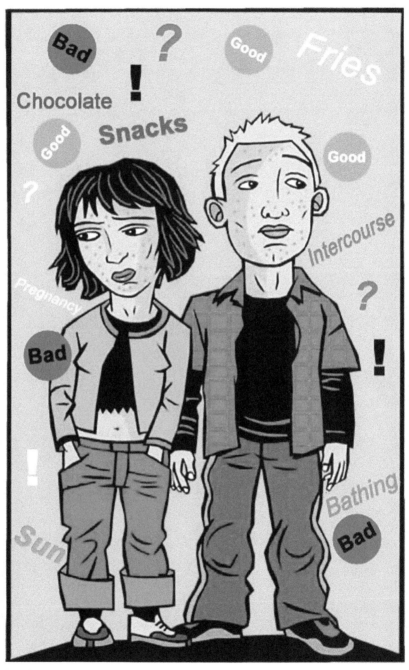

The Acne Solution –

Chapter 11
FOOD AND ITS INFLUENCE ON ACNE

ACNE IN ASSOCIATION WITH DIET

The prevalence of acne in Western populations is around 90% in the majority of the countries. In contrast, acne vulgaris remains rare in non-Western societies. Although familial and ethnic factors are implicated in acne prevalence, the higher incidence rates of acne have increased with the adoption of Western lifestyles.

These observations suggest that lifestyle factors, including diet, may be involved in the implication of acne. Recently, there has been an increasing number of studies investigating the role of diet as one of the underlying causes of acne. Certain dairy products, carbohydrates, highly glycemic-loaded diet that lead to flaring acne support the assumption that what is eaten may affect the skin.

The combination of milk and carbohydrates potentiate insulin hormone levels causing increase androgen hormones that are crucial in acne flare up.

The measurement of glucose (blood sugar) is defined by the "glycemic index." Glycemic index is increased by carbohydrate consumption. This index is less accurate than the measurement of insulin index representing the insulin response (insulin secretion rate). Insulin is a pancreatic hormone secreted as a response to food containing carbohydrates.

Foods with Low Glycemic Index

Legumes such as beans (kidney, white, black, pink, soy); nuts (almonds, peanuts, walnuts, chickpeas), and seeds (sunflower, flax, pumpkin, poppy, sesame); most fruits (peaches, strawberries, mangos), most vegetables (beets, squash, parsnips); most whole grains (durum/spelt/

kamut wheat, millet, oat, rye, rice, barley); fructose.

Foods with Medium Glycemic Index
Cracked whole wheat or enriched wheat; pita bread; basmati rice; potatoes; grape juice; raisins; prunes; pumpernickel bread; cranberry juice; regular ice cream; sucrose.

Foods with High Glycemic Index
White bread (wheat endosperm only); most white rice (rice endosperm only); corn flakes, extruded breakfast cereals; glucose; maltose; potatoes; pretzels.

PROBIOTICS AND THEIR CORRELATION TO ACNE

Probiotics are defined as a dietary supplement containing live bacteria (Example: lactobacilli bacteria) taken orally to restore beneficial effect on human health. Probiotic organisms are live microorganisms that are thought to be beneficial to the host organism.

According to the currently adopted definition by the World Health Organization (WHO), probiotics are "live microorganisms, which when administered in adequate amounts, confer a health benefit on the host."

Ingesting just the right kind of bacteria can exert profound beneficial effects on skin homoeostasis, skin inflammation, hair growth, and peripheral tissue responses to perceived stress.

In those genetically susceptible to acne vulgaris, the cascade presenting excess sebum production, exacerbations in acne and additional psychological distress, both probiotics and antimicrobials may play a role in cutting off this cycle at the gut level.

Probiotics are "generally recognized as safe" (GRAS). This classification is given to products that are composed of ingredients that are natural or have been safely used for many years.

Not all probiotics are created equal. Choose a quality product at the right quantity. Obtain your probiotic from a trusted source. A responsible manufacturer will make sure its probiotic product is potent through to the end of its shelf life as it was in its clinical studies.

Probiotic products are increasingly used by consumers for their health benefits and they are advocated by many healthcare professionals especially in the field of treating acne. The evidence base for their use in specific clinical studies is strong in cases such as acne.

LACTOFERRIN AND ITS BENEFICIAL THERAPEUTIC EFFECT ON ACNE

Lactoferrin is a prominent component of the mucosal defense system whose expression is upregulated in response to inflammatory stimuli. The protein contributes to mammalian host defense by acting as both an antibacterial and anti-inflammatory agent.

Lactoferrin is the second most abundant protein in human milk. Lactoferrin is found in human colostrum. Colostrum is a form of milk produced by the mammary glands of mammals. It contains antibodies to protect the breast-fed infants against bacterial infection, as well as being lower in fat and higher in protein than ordinary milk.

Lactoferrin is a true nutraceutical in that inhibits the development of the bacteria that causes acne and reduces the inflammation associated with existing acne blemishes, working from the inside to help support a healthy completion.

A primary function of Lactoferrin is scavenging free iron in body fluids and inflamed sites to suppress free radical-mediated damage and diminish availability of the element to invading microbes.

A single capsule of (bovine Lactoferrin) 50 mg/day is the suggested dosage as part of regular replenishment for a normal healthy individual. However, depending upon lifestyle, age, and health-status, increasing the dosage to 2-3 capsules per day could benefit certain individuals ingesting fermented milk with 200 mg of Lactoferrin daily for six weeks or fermented milk only for 12 weeks.

Lactoferrin is US FDA approved.

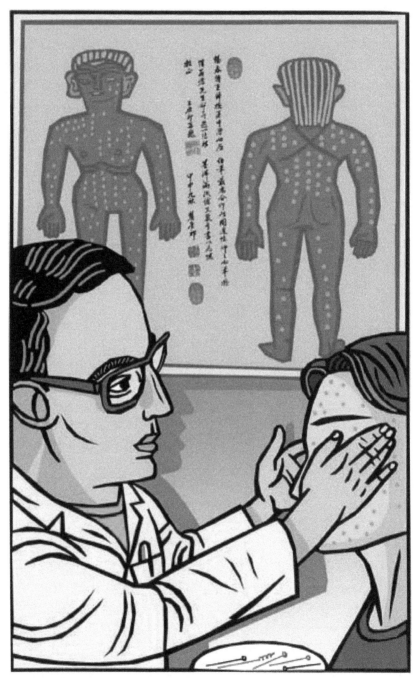

The Acne Solution –

Chapter 12

ACNE AND ALTERNATIVE MEDICINE

At times, skin problems, including acne, respond to some alternative medicine methods, although not all "Western" doctors have faith in these disciplines. Some believe that their success has more to do with mysticism than medicine, while others are convinced that improvement would have taken place in any case, even without treatment.

Nevertheless, in recent years alternative medicine in Israel has become an accepted branch of treatment. Most HMO's have established alternative medicine centers, and similar units also operate in public hospitals.

The decision whether to try one of the types of alternative medicine as a cure for acne must be made by each person individually, in accordance with personal attitudes and experience.

In any case, if this is the road you choose, it would be worthwhile to exercise some personal judgment. Take an interest in the specific field of alternative medicine that you intend to try. Learn more about it, examine the pros and cons of the cure, and inquire about the doctor you are considering. In short, be aware of the effect the treatment might have on you. If you feel that the experience is good for your skin, nothing should keep you from continuing with the treatment.

This chapter does not relate to all areas of alternative medicine, but only to those that may possibly contribute to acne sufferers.

HOMEOPATHY

Homeopathy is the best known of the various alternative medicine treatment methods, as well as the most accepted. Developed in the nineteenth century by Dr. Samuel Hahnemann, it offers more than 4,000 medicines based on natural substances, minerals and various plants.

A homeopath need not be a doctor, but should have homeopathy certification, which requires appropriate training.

What Are the Principles of Homeopathy?
Homeopathy views the manifestations of an illness to be signals of an imbalance in one or more of the body systems. Homeopathic therapy is aimed at restoring the balance.

While Western medicine focuses on the illness or symptom that a patient complains of, homeopathy views the person as a whole. The patient's overall health condition, way of life, personality and worldview are all taken into consideration. The homeopathic therapist will not necessarily propose the same treatment for two different individuals even if they share the same complaint, but will map out an individual treatment for each, according to that patient's particular needs.

One of the basic principles of correct homeopathic theory is assembling an overall picture of the applicant. This stage requires the expertise of an experienced homeopath, and is carried out by means of a comprehensive medical interview.

The fundamental principle on which the method is based is "similar heals similar" ("homeo" in Greek: similar, equal), namely: a substance that can produce symptoms of an illness in a healthy person will cure, in diluted form, the same symptoms in an ill person. The homeopathic therapist believes that the more dilute the medicine, the greater its effect.

The principles of homeopathic therapy are founded on ways of improving the body's self-defense mechanisms, and the body's ability to control the illness. The homeopathic approach assumes that at times a connection exists between the appearance of one illness and the disappearance of another illness, and that the appearance of symptoms of one illness could signal the cure of another illness. For example, a wart could serve as a channel through which asthma can vanish. In such a case, treating the wart may cause a recurrence or aggravation of the asthma for those who suffer from it.

Homeopathy distinguishes between two types of acne and treats each differently:

- Acne in the young is regarded as a natural occurrence in adolescence.
- Acne that begins in adulthood, or carries from adolescence into adulthood. This type of acne is commonly viewed as a reaction of the body to another illness lurking undetected in the body.

Homeopathic treatment of acne uses topical or oral preparations. It may be combined with traditional medications or administered alone.

Treatment may continue for a long time and requires a great deal of patience.

Does It Help?
Success of homeopathic therapy varies from one case to another. At the beginning of the process, the symptoms of the disorder may sometimes worsen, but exactly this reaction may indicate greater chances of successful treatment.

TRADITIONAL CHINESE MEDICINE
The underlying principle of traditional Chinese medicine, as of homeopathy, is to treat the individual as a whole in the existing environment. According to this approach as well, illnesses and various bodily disorders reflect an imbalance in the body.

Outside of China, primarily doctors also qualified in Western medicine practice TCM, so treatment usually integrates both disciplines.

TCM offers two methods for treating acne: acupuncture and Chinese herbal medicine.

Acupuncture

Acupuncture, an ancient Chinese medical discipline, stems from the same traditional Eastern beliefs of healing body and mind together. Acupuncture theory is based on a central concept in Chinese medicine, Qi, the "life force," or energy. The aim of the treatment is to achieve a balance between the equal but opposite energy forces known as Yin and Yang.

According to this concept, the body contains 12 invisible energy pathways called meridians, located on which are hundreds of "critical" points. Various disturbances that block the flow of energy can occur at any of these points. Certain combinations of such disturbances are characteristic of every type of illness. In order to regulate the flow of energy along the blocked pathways and cure the illness, thin needles are inserted at each relevant point.

How Does it Work?

At the first consultation, the acupuncturist strives to learn as much as possible about you and your lifestyle, and then, based on the information obtained, determines the relevant acupuncture points.

Tiny needles are inserted into the skin for a short time, or left in place under supervision for 20 to 30 minutes. Sometimes the therapist burns a mixture of herbs on or near the acupuncture point, removing it when you begin to feel heat. At other times, he may transmit a low electrical current through the needle.

The sensation accompanying the insertion of the needles is described by most people as a moderate tickle, and only rarely as pain.

In recent years, some therapists have taken advantage of lasers by using them at the acupuncture points. This method is especially suited for treating people fearful of needles.

Treatment can be given for very brief periods or continue for several months.

Herbs

Chinese herbal medicine, documented for more than 2,000 years but actually in use for some 4,000 years, treats the cause of the problem or illness and its symptoms.

The doctor or therapist (certified to practice this discipline) will want to be acquainted with your detailed history. He will give you a general examination, examine the color, coating and texture of your tongue, and check the pulse at both your wrists. There are 12 pulses (six on each wrist) related to various areas of the body. They express various imbalances in the system that cause certain syndromes.

After diagnosis, the doctor will give you a prescription consisting of several herbs specifically chosen from a selection of over 160 different herbs. The herbs are used to prepare a tea. At the beginning of the treatment cycle, it is usually recommended to drink one portion of the tea twice daily. As the condition improves, dosage is reduced. Ointments, lotions, rinsing water, compresses, and masks for treating the skin may also be prescribed.

Herbal prescriptions are compounded individually for each patient and are easily adjusted, adding a little of this or removing a little of that. The aim is to first halt the underlying illness, and then improve the condition of the skin until it is completely healed.

After treatment, some people continue to use Chinese herbal medicine as preventive treatment. After their condition improves, they occasionally use an herbal mixture that made for them in order to continue to maintain a healthy skin.

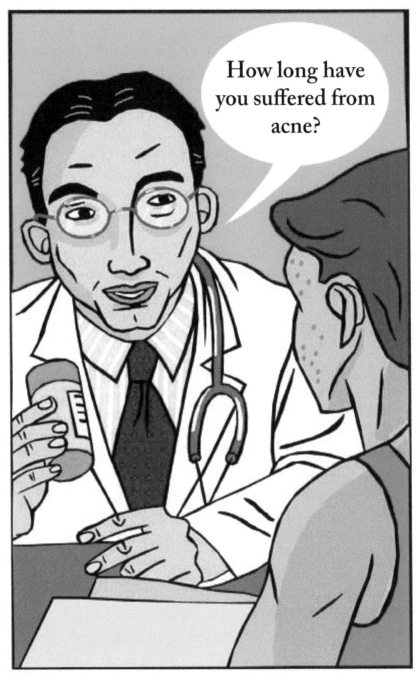

The Acne Solution –

Chapter 13
PARTICULAR TYPES
OF ACNE

Did you know that even an embryo can get zits! Known as prenatal acne, this condition can occur as a result of high levels of androgen hormones in the womb during pregnancy. It disappears a few days after birth.

This of course is a rare occurrence and a distinct type of acne, not the common disorder that takes center stage in this book. Many other types of acne appear at various stages of life.

ACNE IN NEWBORNS

Nursing babies, particularly boys, sometime develop an acne-like rash characterized by small red bumps on the cheeks and forehead. It is thought that the pimples appear as a result of androgen hormones transmitted through nursing from the mother's sebum to the sebaceous glands of the newborn.

The rash requires no treatment and passes within a few months.

Using baby oil on the face and scalp at any age is not recommended since it might aggravate the pimples.

ACNE IN INFANTS AND CHILDREN

This rare form of acne sometimes appears in infants and young children. Generally it goes away by itself within a few weeks or months, although it could last longer, even until adolescence. Whiteheads and blackheads appear on the cheeks and forehead. In rare instances, pustules also appear on the skin, which if not treated, may develop into permanent scars.

Anyone who has suffered from this type of acne in childhood, and if other family members have suffered from ordinary acne, is very likely to suffer severe acne in adolescence. Such children should be under close medical supervision.

Treating acne in infants and children requires maintaining skin cleanliness and applying topical preparations. At times medicinal treatment with antibiotics or vitamins is required.

A child suffering from severe and persistent acne will usually be referred by the doctor for a hormonal examination, first to determine if internal or hormonal disorders are causing the acne.

ACNE FULMINANS (INFLAMED)

Acne Fulminans is a rare, severe and especially difficult form of acne. It appears in adolescent boys and is characterized by inflamed cysts, mostly on the chest and back.

Sometimes the disorder is accompanied by fever, weakness and painful joints. The sores tend to ulcerate and discharge pus.

It is most important to treat this acne urgently, as any delay could cause irreversible damage and permanent scarring. Treatment involves draining the cysts and suppressing the inflammatory process through anti-inflammatory medications such as steroids, and high doses of oral or injected antibiotics.

ACNE IN PREGNANCY

Hormonal changes during pregnancy may in certain cases cause an outbreak of acne, aggravate existing acne, or alternatively, improve its condition.

Treating pimples during pregnancy requires great caution. Topical preparations, or medications harmful to the embryo, must be avoided. The dermatologist should be notified of your pregnancy. It is especially important to check the leaflets included with the various preparations for warnings about taking the medication during pregnancy.

Most medical centers and some health maintenance organizations (HMOs) operate centers that provide information on medications permitted during pregnancy, as well as drug interactions and poisoning. Ask the doctor about the center closest to you.

ACNE IN MIDLIFE

About one-fifth of women over the age of 40 may suffer from midlife acne, even if they have never suffered from acne before. At this stage of life, because a hormonal imbalance may occur due to approaching menopause, or because of cessation of birth control pills, pimples may erupt on the face.

Additional factors (previously mentioned) such as stress and tension, or using various medications or cosmetic preparations that are unsuitable for the skin, may contribute to the outbreak of acne in older age groups, although more in women than in men. Pimples that appear at this stage of life often indicate the presence of various internal disorders.

Appearance of acne in midlife requires medical inquiry to diagnose the background for its appearance. Following this, if no cause is identified, the doctor will usually treat the disorder in the same manner as ordinary acne, with the restrictions dictated by the age and general health of the patient.

ACNE ROSACEA

Rosacea is a skin disorder causing redness, tendency to flushing, swelling and pustules on the face. Unlike ordinary acne, blackheads or whiteheads do not characterize rosacea.

More common in women than men, this disorder usually appears in women aged 30 to 50, and only in exceptional cases in younger women as well.

People under stress and tension are more inclined to suffer from this disorder.

Identifying Signs

The typical redness of rosacea usually appears in the central part of the face, spreading at the more advanced stages to the forehead, nose, cheeks and chin. As it progresses, blood vessels in the area dilate. Pustules form, and more rarely, small reddish-brown pimples as well. At times additional signs appear, such as disturbances of the digestive system, inflammation and a burning sensation in the eyes, oily skin, and scalp dandruff.

In acute cases of this disorder, particularly among men, the nose may swell to twice its natural size. This occurrence can be clearly seen among serious drinkers.

If you see such indications on face, see your dermatologist immediately. Without treatment, rosacea progresses and becomes more severe. It may even cause permanent damage to your skin.

Before making a diagnosis, the dermatologist will determine

if internal disorders are producing symptoms similar to those of rosacea.

Aggravating Factors

Rosacea sufferers must avoid all factors that increase blood flow to the face, and contribute to flushing, swelling or irritation of facial skin. Note in particular the following guidelines:

- Avoid drinking alcoholic or hot beverages, consuming strong spices, and smoking.
- Avoid exposure to the sun and make certain to use sunscreen lotions.
- Avoid extreme and rapid transitions from heat to cold and vice versa.
- Avoid cosmetic massages and skin peeling treatment in the area of the redness.
- Avoid, as much as possible, situations of stress and tension. These too cause congestion in facial blood vessels.
- Avoid using hair sprays and other substances that irritate the skin.
- Avoid using cosmetic preparations that irritate your face.

Treating Rosacea

In mild cases, ointments containing metronidazole (Rosax, for example) are applied. These are effective in treating the inflammatory component of rosacea, but have no effect on the dilated facial blood vessels.

In more severe cases, the doctor will prescribe lengthy antibiotic treatment with tetracycline or minocycline, sometimes with the addition Flagyl (when deeper infections must be suppressed).

In very severe cases of the disorder, when the skin is especially red and inflamed, the doctor may recommend treatment with Roaccutane/Accutane. The inflammatory component responds well to treatment with this medication, and it can considerably reduce the redness.

Vitamin B can be integrated in the treatment, for its potential for reducing excretions of the sebaceous glands. Take note: in certain cases, the vitamin can cause blushing of facial skin, in which case, it should, of course, be stopped at once.

Dilated blood vessels and redness are treated most successfully with dedicated laser devices, operating on the appropriate wavelength. The laser beam burns and clears the dilated vessels.

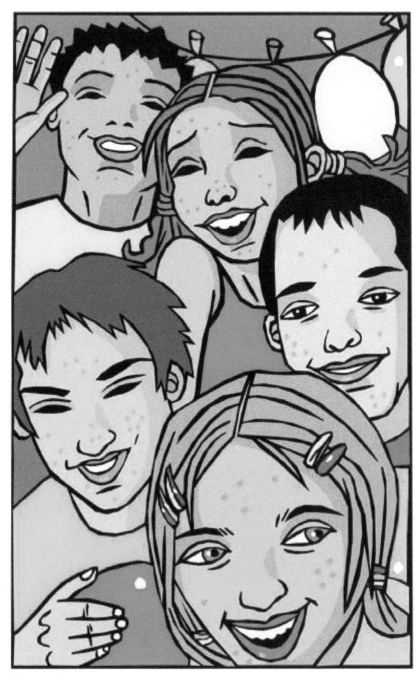

The Acne Solution –

Chapter 14
ACNE AND YOUR MOOD

Acne does not only affect the appearance of your face, but most likely, at least to some extent, you also feel its effect on your mood. Let's look a little at a subject we often tend to ignore: the mental and social difficulties that may accompany acne.

Appearance has an important function in interpersonal relationships. Fresh, smooth skin projects vitality and good health. Acne – being so visible and difficult to conceal mars the appearance of your skin. It is natural to be apprehensive that this may adversely affect social attitudes toward you. This fear of rejection in some cases activates a destructive chain reaction: your self-image is undermined, you're reluctant and more hesitant to form social relationships, more inclined to isolate yourself, and so on and on...

WHY, OF ALL TIMES, DURING ADOLESCENCE?

The timing of the appearance of acne – of all times during adolescence– is particularly problematic. At this age the changes taking place in the body are the external expression of sexual development: with boys, their voices become deeper and they begin to shave; girls buy their first bra and begin to menstruate. Everything is new, different, turbulent, and you become more sensitive as well as more vulnerable.

This is the time when you examine your appearance as an adult. More than ever, you look at yourself in the mirror, adopt role models for emulation, compare yourself with your peers and crave positive reinforcements approving your appearance. Also, this is the time when you may experience your first romantic relationship.

And then, just then, pimples erupt and wreak havoc on your face. No wonder that this is a difficult crisis for so many of you, marked by feelings of frustration and anger, often causing you to dump blame on yourself and everyone around you.

LEARN TO ACCEPT YOURSELF FOR WHO YOU ARE: NOT PERFECT

We live in a competitive world that encourages excellence and perfection in all areas of life, and above all, in our external appearance. You, just like all of us, see all around you gorgeous models, beautiful actors, muscular athletes – all tall and perfect, with smooth and glowing skin. The cosmetics and makeup industries promise to make you flawless, if you only continue to use the preparations they market. The hidden message being constantly transmitted to you is that once you get that new look, you'll be able to achieve anything you want.

No one in the cosmetics illusion industry will tell you that the "perfect" appearance of models as seen in the advertising shots, is most often achieved only by special lighting, utilizing flattering camera angles, and the hours-long application of makeup. Photographs also undergo a process of retouching and refinishing that give the models their astonishing and very enviable appearance.

It's important to say to yourself again and again that you are not perfect, and there is no one definition of external beauty. Every one of you has a personality that is special and different, and a unique appearance. We all must learn to accept ourselves as we are. Good and effective treatment of your skin, and concealing pimples and scars, is the correct way to improve your appearance and self-image. You should try to appear as pleasant, well groomed, and esthetic as possible, but try not to make this the focal point of your life.

Investing in beauty and inner richness leads to a feeling of satisfaction and personal and social achievements for each and every one of us.

COPE! DON'T BLAME THE PIMPLES

Among your friends are probably those who go "nuts" over a single pimple, and those who remain unperturbed with a face full of zits. The difference between them stems from their attitude toward themselves. People who are comfortable with themselves do not tend to blame their difficulties on pimples, and cope with them in the same way they cope with any other medical problem. On the other hand, those who are unsure of themselves and most affected by reactions from the surroundings, get stressed out every time a little pimple appears. Among them, you will always find those who blame pimples for destroying their social relationships.

But there really is no point in blaming acne for the state of your social life. An "uneven floor" can't be blamed every time you fall. Better to learn to recognize the real reasons for your problems, to learn how to dance.

PIMPLES ARE JUST TEMPORARY

Imagine yourself a driving a car, trying to reach the destination you set for yourself through force of willpower, persistence and with the help of your surroundings. The appearance of pimples is like suddenly getting a flat: it interrupts travel, wastes time and irritates, but it can be fixed. No one changes their car because of a flat tire! This is how you have to relate to your acne. You must be patient and persistent and remember that most acne patients recover within a reasonable time. You must think positively, and enlist your resources for fighting the pimples and the frustrations.

YOU DESERVE PROPER TREATMENT - DON'T RELY ON MIRACLES AND RUMORS

One reason for the many frustrations is listening to old wives' tales and trying treatment methods that contribute nothing to improving the condition. You will always be surrounded by "advisers" who have tried every possible treatment of acne, except for the treatment that is appropriate for them. They will tell you that treatment doesn't help and will lead you into despair.

Don't rely on prophets and doomsayers. Professionals – cosmeticians, dermatologists, and if necessary, psychologists can guide you to the solution of your problem. Why not go to them? Doing this will substantially shorten the length of treatment, contribute to your emotional wellbeing, and prevent unnecessary frustration.

ACNE IS ONLY ACNE – NO MORE

Acne, as conspicuous as it may seem, is only a very small factor in your life. Allowing this one element, unpleasant as it may be, to detract from your happiness and complicate your social relationships, is totally unreasonable. Acne is not the "end of the world," and there is no connection whatsoever between it and your skills and abilities. Does a manager succeed only because of perfect face skin? Will an outstanding soldier with pimples be rejected for training with the Navy SEALs because of pimples?

You must relate to your body skin as external wrapping. Even if the wrapping has a few defects and flaws, the internal contents remain intact. What would you rather get for your birthday: a valuable present wrapped in inexpensive paper, or a worthless present wrapped in expensive paper?

It would be wise to remember an old saying, "don't judge a book by its cover..."

Glossary

ACNE VULGARIS
The Latin name of the common form of acne mostly affecting adolescents. Commonly known as "pimples" or "zits."

ANDROGENS
A group of male sex hormones produced mainly in the testes. These hormones are produced to a lesser extent in women's ovaries.

BLACKHEAD
Oily sebum plug. When exposed to air, it oxidizes and turns black. Commonly appears in the areas of the nose, cheeks, and chin.

COLLAGEN
A protein that naturally occurs in skin connective tissue, cartilage and bones. It is one of the most commonly used materials in Western medicine for filling scars and repairing esthetic blemishes.

COMEDO
Latin name for blackhead or whitehead (plural: comedones).

CYSTS
Large red sacs, usually filled with fluid, formed under the skin when pores become completely clogged. This is the most severe stage in the inflammatory process. Cysts may leave scars on the skin.

DERMIS
Middle layer of the skin, under the epidermis. Consists of an elastin and collagen fiber base, networks of blood vessels, sebaceous glands, sweat glands, nerve endings, and hair follicles.

EPIDERMIS
External skin layer. Rough on its outer surface due to dead skin cells which accumulate before shedding.

ESTROGEN
One of two female hormones produced in the ovaries. Governs secondary sexual characteristics. Estrogen is produced in much smaller quantities in the male testes.

GLYCEMIC INDEX

An index that provides a measure of how quickly blood sugar levels (i.e., levels of glucose in the blood) rise after eating a particular type of food. The effects that different foods have on blood sugar levels vary considerably. The glycemic index estimates how much each gram of available carbohydrate (total carbohydrate minus fiber) in a food raises a person's blood glucose level following consumption of the food, relative to consumption of pure glucose. Glucose has a glycemic index of 100.

HAIR FOLLICLE

A tubular structure in the skin containing the hair shaft through which the hair grows to the skin surface

HORMONES

Mediating chemical substances produced by the body for regulating almost all body functions.

INFLAMMATION

Reaction of body tissues to infection, immune system disorder, or injury.

KERATIN

Tough insoluble protein manufactured by cells rising to the outer skin layer. Keratin is also found in hair, teeth, and nails.

KERATIN PLUG

A plug that forms within the hair follicle, causing it to clog. Composed of thousands of dead skin cells, loaded with a tough insoluble protein (keratin), stuck to each with sebum, hair particles, bacteria and their byproducts.

LACTOFERRIN

A multifunctional protein that is one of the components of the immune system of the body; it has antimicrobial activity (bactericide, fungicide) that inhibits the development of the bacteria that causes acne.

LASER BEAM

A concentrated coherent beam of light with unique properties. Used in medicine for performing surgical procedures requiring pinpoint accuracy, as well as for cutting and fusing body tissues.

PAPULE

An inflamed pimple seen as a small red bump. It's the body's reaction to the sebum ejected from a whitehead into adjoining tissues that reject it as a foreign body.

PHOTOTHERAPY

Light therapy directed at the skin is also used to treat acne. It consists of exposure to specific wavelengths of light using polychromatic polarised light, lasers, light-emitting diodes, fluorescent lamps, dichroic lamps or very bright, full-spectrum light, usually controlled with various devices. The light is administered for a prescribed amount of time and, in some cases, at a specific time of day.

PROBIOTICS

Probiotics are live bacteria taken orally to restore beneficial effect on human health. Some strains may modulate the inflammatory and hyper-sensitivity responses of acne sufferers.

PROGESTERONE

One of two female hormones produced by the ovaries that prepares the reproductive system for pregnancy.

PROPIONIBACTERIUM ACNES (P. ACNES)

The bacterium that causes acne. Located on the skin surface, it feeds on the sebum secreted onto the skin. The bacteria break up sebum into fatty acids, which in turn damage the sebum ducts and the hair follicle, a situation that ultimately leads to inflammatory acne.

PUS

Viscous substance, composed of dead white cells, tissue and bacteria remnants. Pus accumulates in an infected wound when the immune system responds to an attack by foreign bodies.

PUSTULE

A papule containing pus-filled liquid. Severe form of acne indicating the presence of inflammation and infection.

SCAR, CRATER-LIKE

Sunken scar: concave, rounded, relatively shallow, sometimes with raised edges.

SCAR, HYPERTROPHIC
Raised, puffy scar

SCAR, KELOID
Raised, puffy scar extending beyond the affected area

SEBACEOUS GLAND
Gland attached to the hair follicle that produces sebum, used to lubricate the skin and hair.

SEBUM
An oily substance produced in the skin by the sebaceous glands. Its function is to lubricate the skin and hair.

SEX HORMONES
Hormones governing sexual development and functioning of the reproductive system. In women, two sex hormones, estrogen and progesterone, are produced in the ovaries. In men, the male sex hormone testosterone is produced in the testes.

SUBCUTANEOUS TISSUE
The innermost layer of the skin, composed of fatty cells. Separates the internal parts of the body from the two external layers of the skin it supports.

TESTOSTERONE
Male sex hormone produced in the testes. This hormone is present in women as well, but in much smaller quantities.

WHITEHEAD
Closed, oily plug appearing just under the skin surface as a small white or skin colored bump

ACNE ON THE WEB
Much effort is being invested today in treating acne. The Internet enables us to keep abreast of the latest innovations, view photographs and illustrations that describe the development of blemishes, and to consult frequently with dermatologists as well as share experiences with other adolescents. It is important to ascertain that the sites visited are objective and provide tested and balanced information rather than exclusively supported by a particular product or manufacturer. More information can be found on the **American Academy of Dermatology website: http://www.aad.org/,** as well as on the **American Acne and Rosacea Society website: http://www.acneandrosacea.org/site.php.**

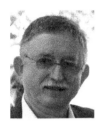

ZEEV PAM, M.D. was born in 1953 in Warsaw, Poland. At the age of four, Zeev and his family immigrated to Israel as members of the cooperative farming settlement Misgav Dov. Married to Sarah Pam and father to two sons, Ori and Nadav Pam, he graduated from the Technion Faculty of Medicine in 1978 and served as a doctor in the IDF. He specialized in dermatology and venereology at Rambam Health Care Campus, Haifa, and from 1991-2013, he was the CEO of Aripam Medical Center, Ashdod, Israel, which was one of the busiest private clinics in southern Israel. In 2010, he founded Derma Pam Ltd., an Israeli pharmaceutical company.

Dr. Pam had many years of clinical experience specializing in hair loss, food supplements, cosmetology, and phototherapy. He was a member of the Israeli Dermatological Society and the American Academy of Dermatology. Dr. Pam passed away 20.01.2013.

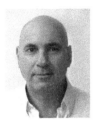

SHMUEL YORAV, M.D. was born in 1955 in Tel Aviv.
He is married to Orna Yorav and the father of two sons, Roy and On Yorav. After graduating from the Tel Aviv University School of Medicine, he served as a medical commanding officer in the IDF. Specializing in dermatology, cosmetic dermatology, laser treatment, and phototherapy for acne. Dr. Yorav is a senior physician in SHEBA Medical Center Tel Hashomer Hospital ,and has a private clinic in Tel Aviv. He is a member of the The Israeli Society of Dermatology and Venereology and the Israeli Society for Dermatological Surgery. As well as a member of the American and European Academies of Dermatology. He is a pharmaceutical consultant as well.

For further information please contact:
www.dryorav.co.il
yorav.md@gmail.com

www.ingramcontent.com/pod-product-compliance
Lightning Source LLC
Jackson TN
JSHW071340130125
77033JS00027B/1004